THE CLASSICAL HOMŒOPATHIC
LECTURES OF

Dr. Med. Vassilis G H E G A S

VOLUME A

May 1987
Bloemendaal (NL)

HOMEO-STUDY v.z.w.
De Schom 67, B-3600 GENK
BELGIUM

This book contains information, given by Dr. Med. Vassilis GHEGAS during the seminar of May 1987 in Bloemendaal (NL). This seminar was organized by the "School voor Homeopathie" (NL).

Written and worked out by **Fons VANDEN BERGHE**

Correction: **Vassilis GHEGAS**

Translation and lay-out: **Roel STRZEMINSKI**

Proof reading: **Deborah COLLINS (NL)**
Frank PICCART (B)
Richard WYNNE (GB)

Design cover and logo: **Brita STRZEMINSKI**

Published by: **HOMEO-STUDY v.z.w.**
De Schom 67
B-3600   GENK
BELGIUM

ISBN 90-74077-14-5
D/1991/6124/3
Reprinted 1994

GENERAL PREFACE

Vassilis GHEGAS was born in Greece in 1948.

During his medical studies, he came in contact with George VITHOULKAS who aroused his interest in classical homœopathy. He started to specialize after obtaining his medical degree, but after a while he left the hospital to study homœopathy with George VITHOULKAS at the Athenian School for Homœopathy.

Vassilis GHEGAS was one of the first and best students at the Athenian School, and he also took an active part in the organization. He has been treating his patients exclusively homœopathically since 1974, first in his teacher's centre and during the latter years in his own practice.

Since 1984, he has given international seminars, first in London (England) and later also in the Netherlands, Germany etc.

From 1987 to 1989, he started a systematic course, organized by the School for Homœopathy in Bloemendaal, Holland. The course has been continued from 1989 to 1992, but this time organized by the "Stichting Homeopathische Opleidingen (S.H.O.)" in Wageningen, Holland.

In these particularly didactic and systematic seminars, Vassilis gives us an enormous diversity of subjects from homœopathic practice:

- Essences of the polychrests
- Smaller remedies and their main fields of application
- How a first or second consultation should be, how to handle homœopathic patients

- Remedies in children
- Philosophy: how does Homœopathy work?
- Discussion of clinical chapters: fears, sexuality, asthma, traumas, pregnancy etc.
- Differential diagnosis of rubrics from the Repertory
- Long-term constitutional treatment
- Serious acute situations where you are obstructed with constitutional remedies
- Obstructed cases
- Etc.

As regards content, it can be noticed that Vassilis has assimilated his teacher's 25-year experience and that he has meticulously tested everything by his own practice.
In his seminars, he only puts forward things he learned from his own experience. His information is very practically- and patient-oriented. He always succeeds in finding a new point of view to consider the patients' problems in order to come to a homœopathic solution.

The didactic qualities of Vassilis are really unique: he puts forward a very complicated matter in a simple way, so that it is practicable and comprehensible to everyone.
One of his best qualities is his sense of putting things in hierarchical order. Therefore, he uses the following experiences:

- What will occur most in practice?
- Which remedies are for a certain problem of first, second or third degree?
- Which symptoms are exclusively characteristic of one, particular remedy and exclude all others?
- Etc.

With all this, it is remarkable how meticulously Vassilis follows the Materia Medica of James Tyler KENT and William BOERICKE, and how he plays with the Repertory of Kent.

Every single lecture of Vassilis GHEGAS is highly recommended to be heard "live": each lecture complements another, his style of teaching is very typical, humorous and surprising, and his simple English is understandable to non-native speakers.
Progressively, the level of his seminars will become more difficult

and of a higher degree. In order to fully understand Vassilis, it is necessary to study his previous information and it is recommended to have some years of practice to make maximum use of his information.

In order to maintain the knowledge provided by Vassilis and to make it of practical use, we conceived the idea of recording all his lectures on the basis of our own notes, combined with existing audiotapes.

At the moment, more than 10 Dutch and English seminars are written down in Dutch. These are now one by one being translated into English, while Vassilis corrects them.

Looking up information from all the books will be made easy by making a comprehensive index by remedy, subject or clinical rubric, as in the Dutch. In this way, you can find at a single glance where Vassilis told something about a certain remedy or subject in his seminars.

To make it easier for inexperienced homœopaths, who are not familiar with the Materia Medica or the Repertory, references to the following most used works have been inserted:

-   The Repertory of the Materia Medica by James Tyler KENT.
-   The Homœopathic Materia Medica by William BOERICKE.
-   The additions in KENT's Repertory by George VITHOULKAS, written down by Bill Gray in 1979.

I hope you will find pleasure in reading and studying these volumes! I also hope that, with you too, the application of information from the Athenian School will lead to better results in practice!

Fons Vanden Berghe

P.S. Remarks, corrections and suggestions are always welcome at the editor's address.

CONTENTS

PREFACE TO VOLUME A

In this first seminar, Vassilis discusses the <u>essence of NAT-M., NAT-S. and SULPH.</u>

Besides, he gives a lot of information about <u>treatment of acute diseases</u> in daily homœopathic practice. You might get the impression that in acute diseases you have to look for remedies used for these acute diseases. But nothing is further from the truth!

Vassilis underlines again and again that in a classic homœopathic consultation you always have to take a complete homœopathic history of the patient and to look for the polychrest that is most suited for the patient in general (Information about the homœopathic consultation will be discussed in detail in future volumes).

If a remedy is perfect for a patient, in essence, keynotes or in its totality, you have to give this remedy, without regard to the complaint which brought the patient to you (Mostly, it will concern a polychrest).

If however, the whole does not correspond to a specific remedy, you have to look for the <u>specific homœopathic remedy that corresponds to the specific acute situation</u> (This can be a polychrest or a small remedy).

From the experiences of the Athenian School and from his own experiences, Vassilis summarizes hierarchically the remedies indicated in one, specific acute situation, such as:

- Common cold
- Tonsillitis
- Whooping cough and severe cough
- Gastritis
- Cystitis
- Colitis and diarrhœa
- Allergic rhinitis
- Skin disorders
- Acne on the face
- Cancer
- Headache

Bear in mind that the use of this information in classical homœopathy is only justified if there is no other constitutional remedy indicated, or if your constitutional treatment is obstructed while your patient is developing a serious acute disease. In such cases, using this information will often help you so that the patient will not need antibiotics or other allopathic medication, and he will not turn his back on homœopathic treatment.

Fons Vanden Berghe
February 1992

THE NATRUMS : ESSENCE

ALL NATRUMS ARE HYPER-SENSITIVE AND CLOSED

To suppress their hypersensitivity in this difficult world, they sometimes start using alcoholic drinks, tranquillizers and even drugs like marihuana and heroin.

The central idea with all NATRUMS is:

INJURY

NAT-M. : injury on the emotional level

NAT-S. : injury on the physical level

NAT-C. : injury on the emotional and the mental level

Here, Vassilis will give the essence of 4 NATRUMS in decreasing frequency of occurrence:

- NATRUM-MURIATICUM: is most frequently found.
- NATRUM-SULPHURICUM
- NATRUM-CARBONICUM: see next volume.
- NATRUM PHOSPHORICUM: see next volume.

NATRUM MURIATICUM : ESSENCE

The central idea of **NAT-M.** is:

> ## INJURY ON THE EMOTIONAL PLANE

With NAT-M., you will nearly always find a number of events in their life that have seriously injured them.

Sometimes, you can find several IGNATIA-experiences or a succession of several IGN. experiences.

To be injured so seriously on the emotional plane, NAT-M. has to be very sensitive.

They are very understanding people: they understand others with problems very well because they have known themselves a lot of problems. That's why it seems that everybody with problems will talk to NAT-M. They feel NAT-M. understands them and they know that NAT-M. won't talk.

NAT-M. will protect and shield himself in order not to be injured all the time: they are introverted: they build a wall round themselves and withdraw behind it. The more others come to talk about their problems, the more introverted NAT-M. becomes. They hear new experiences of how one can be injured and they will try to pretect themselves against it. They are locked up in themselves and have no communication with others anymore.

NAT-M. knows very well when he can be injured and by whom. They will avoid these situations and these persons and they withdraw.

1. HOW TO RECOGNIZE THE CENTRAL IDEA IN NAT-M.

NAT-M. IS A PERFECTIONIST

NAT-M. wants not to be criticized so as not to be injured. That's why they try not to make faults. They are perfectionists, try to do everything perfectly because they can't bear someone seeing their faults. You can add NAT-M. 2nd degree with "fastidious" (K. p. 42) (d.d. NUX-V. is a perfectionist because of his ambitions).

NAT-M. IS VERY CONTROLLED

NAT-M.-patients themselves are easily injured and they think that everyone is easily injured. They avoid everything that might injure others: they check and control themselves. That's why they sometimes reach for medication or alcohol.

- They are polite and friendly. They never speak badly of others. They don't tease, don't make jokes. They are serious (K. p. 55: indifference, pleasure, to).
- They are silent. He who talks a lot can easily injure and this is what they try to avoid. They may remarkably become talkative and less controled after alcohol or wine.

- They have <u>persistent thoughts</u> (K. p. 87: thoughts, unpleasant subjects, haunted by). Every night, they check the past day: have I injured anyone today? If they said too much, they feel guilty. They can be sleepless because of those persistent thoughts about several unpleasant things from the past (K. p. 39: dwells on past disagreeable occurrences). Sometimes, it looks like a "happy melancholy": they worry and worry, which makes them feel very unhappy, but yet don't want to stop it.
- They are sometimes <u>very passive</u>. They sometimes prefer to do nothing than start something which might hurt others.

NAT-M. IS VERY OBJECTIVE

NAT-M. is a good observer and <u>they understand without a word everybody round them</u> and everything that happens round them. Because of their closeness, they stay as it were out of the occurrences and the feelings of others. This makes them good <u>objective observers</u>.

E.g.: A female NAT-M. goes with her husband to a party. She doesn't talk a lot but has seen and felt everything. Afterwards, she will be able to say of all the people her husband had spoken to if they had honest intentions or not and if they lied or not, and mostly she is right.
If at the same party however, someone draws the attention to her, she will be frightened, get a red colour and lose her objective observation. Then, she thinks this person has the same as she has and that this person understands her.

NAT-M. IS VERY KIND AND DOESN'T GET ANGRY

If something negative happens, they are easily hurt and grieved (K. p. 50: grief; K. p. 51:ailments from; grief, silent). They won't tell anybody but will be plunged into worry. They think: you did so much for that person, and now he/she is so ungrateful. NAT-M. never forgets what has happened, unpleasant things will be remembered for years.

If NAT-M. has a discussion with someone and they think they have hurt him/her, they may call afterwards to ask if he/she is alright, without telling the reason why they are calling. They feel easily GUILTY.

DURING THE INTERVIEW, NAT—M. IS MOSTLY CLOSED

They keep everything to themselves. The patient is very serious. As a therapist, you get the impression that the patient has already solved his problems. This may make you feel bored and inferior, even if the patient has serious troubles. When you, as a therapist, call a NAT-M.-patient from the waiting room, you can sometimes see they are shy because you say their name loud and clear. When you then ask their name in the consultation, you will get a cautious answer. If you ask their phone number, they might answer: "Is this really necessary?". Sometimes they say: "My family doesn't know I'm here, I'm here in private."

Sometimes, there is no good communication with NAT-M. during the interview. You may get the impression that they need something from you and that they will pay for it.

D.d. NAT-C.:

With them, there is good cooperation and communication. They will try to help you find their remedy. You won't get the feeling they need something from you. They are always smiling. When you ask them if they are always so happy, they will answer: "No, not internally."

NAT-M. SELDOM WEEPS IN THE CONSULTATION ROOM

A NAT-M.-patient rarely shows his grief. If a patient weeps at the beginning of the interview, it can hardly be NAT-M. (K. p. 51: grief, ailments from, cannot cry).
If you fire your questions one after the other, a NAT-M.-patient will become even more suspicious and closed.
If you want to know more details, they'll try to shield themselves. Then, at a certain moment, you may get the impression that the patient regrets coming to you. You may get the impression they want to stop the interview and want to go out.

If however, you have good contact with the NAT-M.-patient and they have the feeling you understand them, that you recognize their problems, and that you are looking for a solution, they will be more and more open and give more and more information. If NAT-M. tells about deep grief, they may exceptionally burst out in hysterical, loud crying with enormous power. It looks as if all their grief, held for years, suddenly explodes. Afterwards, the therapist can feel guilty because he made the patient cry.

If you have exceptionally good contact with NAT-M., they are very loyal afterwards: they need your help, your friendship and affection and you are the only one who understands them.

NAT-M. IS EASILY DISSAPOINTED IN LOVE

NAT-M. can suffer a lot after the end of a love affair or after a divorce (K. p. 63: love, ailments from disappointed, with silent grief). They love their partner very much, but expect a lot in exchange for it. If the expectations are not fulfilled, the relationship may easily break and once again, NAT-M. is INJURED.
If NAT-M. has been injured several times or disappointed in relationships, they will easily fall in love platonically. They only try to love mentally, not physically, e.g. with someone they will never meet. They thus hope to spare themselves the next "grief".

E.g.: A girl who was in love with a singer. Every night, she listened to his music. She said: "His music dances in me, his voice is in resonance with my inner being."

D.d. NAT-C.: Are less disappointed in love: they love their partner very much, but give themselves completely; they don't expect anything back.

NAT–M. LIKES SOFT MUSIC

They feel happy with soft music. They can't dance in public, but internally, they dance to the music.

Other remedies that are sensitive to music are:
- AUR.
- NAT-C.: music gives an emotional amelioration.
- GRAPH.: weeps with music.
- NAT-S.: music gives an emotional amelioration.
- TARENT.: music gives a physical amelioration, it calms them.

2. THE NAT-M.-CHILD

- They are introverted, closed, have no or few friends.
- They learn to speak late and with difficulty (K. p. 86: talk, slow, learning to). To protect themselves against faults, they stop their efforts at learning to speak. They sometimes also learn late to walk (K. p. 1223: extremities, walk, late, learning to). They sometimes walk in their sleep (K. p. 81: somnambulism).

- They have a pale face, with a very soft skin which gives the idea that it could easily tear. They are often slender and look delicate. Especially the neck and chest can be slender (K. p. 887: back, emaciation, cervical region).
- Sometimes, a horizontal line can be seen in the lower or upper eyelid. This line can also be seen with other hysterical remedies like ASAF., MOSCH., LIL-T.
- They are good students at school, but they say nothing, they are very quiet and silent. If the teacher asks them something, they can give a perfect answer and everybody is surprised about their knowledge. In the play time, they sit in a corner or on the toilet. After school, they immediately go home. At home, they won't tell anything about school.
- They need much love and affection from their parents, but the parents can't get contact with their child and say: "My child is cold on the emotional plane." In their grief, they don't want to be disturbed (K. p. 16: consolation agg.). They feel every disharmony in their environment, between their own parents as well as in other families.
- If you come into contact with a NAT-M.-child, you mostly don't give much affection because the child is so serious, closed and introverted. This causes the child to be even more introverted and this causes a viscious circle.
- They like music and books. They mostly read a lot of books.

3. THE NAT-M.-ADOLESCENT

- They are very intelligent, competent, kind and friendly. Yet, they are closed, introverted and serious. The reaction of others is mostly to keep some distance from youngsters who are too serious. Inside, they believe they deserve friendship and appreciation of others. As they do not always get this, they become more introverted. Here, we get the same as with AURUM.

- NAT-M.-youngsters like to be alone. When they go to a party, they sit silently in a corner. They observe everything, have seen everything round them. If someone asks them to dance, they will be shy. They think everyone is watching them while they are dancing. Afterwards, they often go to the toilet to be alone for a minute.
- NAT-M.-youngsters understand the others without one single word. They know if the parents had a quarrel, and understand every row. If the parents want a divorce, they will be very sad, and melancholic. If one of the parents then asks what is wrong, they won't answer unless they insist, and then they will say: "I'm sure you're going to divorce."
  If the parents will divorce, the child can have spasms or cry hysterically. Mostly, the school results will decline.
  They may react hysterically if you want to console them.

4. CHARACTERISTIC MENTAL SYMPTOMS OF NAT-M. AND THEIR D.D.

NAT-M. LIKES TO BE ALONE

(K. p. 12: company, aversion to)

- BAR-C.: they are childish and they know it. They think everybody will laugh at them and for that reason they won't come out.

- GELS.: are too weak, they will lose more energy in a group.

- IGN.: are afraid that someone will remind them of their problem and that they will react hysterically while others are watching.

- NAT-M.: are afraid to be hurt in a group.

- NUX-V.: will easily have a discussion or argue in a group.

NAT-M. DOESN'T WANT COMPANY DURING URINATION

(K. p. 12: company, aversion to, presence of strangers, during urination)

- You will find this symptom with NAT-M. in 8 out of 10 cases.
- In order to find this symptom, you could ask them what they would do if they have to go urgently while they are walking in a park or a wood. NAT-M. will certainly wait till they have found a toilet. In a wood, they will go very far until no one can see them anymore.
- A NAT-M.-man in a public toilet will do as if he has to make stool and urinate in a closed W.C.
- When a NAT-M.-patient is hospitalized, everybody has to leave the room when they have to urinate or to make stool (d.d. AMBRA GRISEA).

NAT-M. DOESN'T WANT TO TALK IN A GROUP AND DOESN'T WANT TO BE CONSOLED

(K. p. 16: conversation agg.; consolation agg.)

- <u>IGN.</u>: in case of problems, they are so busy with themselves that they won't hear what you say or don't pay attention to you. They are as it were in another world. The consolation has no effect and you have to stop it.

- <u>LIL-T.</u>: they go away, close the door with a smash so that it bursts and cry: "Leave me alone!"

- <u>NAT-M.</u>: is more serious, they ask kindly: "Would you please leave me alone now?"

- <u>SEP.</u>: is more ironical and sarcastic, will laugh with you and hurt you because you want to console them (spiteful). They say: "You're naïve, do you want to console me? Look at yourself!"

- <u>SIL.</u> will calmly explain to you: "I'm too tired now and a bit confused, so shall we go on later?"

NAT–M. IS EASILY DISAPPOINTED IN LOVE

(K. p. 63: love, ailments from disappointed)

- <u>IGN.</u>: likes to be in company and behaves hysterically.

- <u>PULS.</u>: can't stop weeping.

- <u>PH-AC.</u>: becomes in such situations very indifferent and weak, especially emotionally, but later also physically and mentally.

- <u>NAT-M.</u>: they don't want to see anybody and they lock themselves up in the acute phase.

NAT–M. SUFFERS TERRIBLY FROM MORTIFICATIONS

(K. p. 68: mortification, ailments after)

- <u>COLOC.</u>: they get pain in stomach or abdomen and have to bend double.

- <u>IGN.</u>: reacts hysterically.

- STAPH.: they suppress themselves in order not to react and remain silent.

- NAT-M.: they are irritable, can't express themselves. They start worrying at night in bed: they think of everything beyond all proportion and can't sleep all night. They even worry about all similar situations in the past. They talk to themselves, blame themselves and even swear at themselves.

- PH-AC.: becomes indifferent to everything. They get very weak on the emotional plane (K. p. 55: indifference, everything, to).

NAT-M. IS EASILY OFFENDED

(K. p. 69: offended, easily)

- NUX-V.: they are easily beside themselves with rage and this can make them start crying.

- NAT-M.: can be added 3rd degree in this rubric. NAT-M. is easily angry but won't say anything, they can't express themselves.

NAT-M. IS SYMPATHETIC

(K. p. 86: sympathetic)

You have to ask the patient for examples to read this symptom, so you can better form your opinion.

- PHOS.: goes where the problem is, offers help, and will even accompany an injured person to the hospital.

- NAT-M.: they don't want others to see they are sympathetic. They are too shy to go where the problem is. They can become depressed from sympathy.

5. AFFECTION OF NAT-M. BY SUCCESSIVE EMOTIONAL INJURIES

A. PHYSICAL PROBLEMS

NAT-M. has a strong defense system. That's why they first only show physical symptoms, such as:

- headaches
- herpes round the lips
- ulcers and gastritis
- heart palpitations
- affections of the thyroid gland
- neurological diseases such as multiple sclerosis

B. MENTAL-EMOTIONAL PROBLEMS

If the affection gets deeper and deeper, NAT-M. will also show mental-emotional troubles after a long time:

- melancholy, with masochistic ideas on the emotional plane. Women can be very melancholic before or during the menses and yet not weep (K. p. 77: sadness, menses, before).

- irritability: there can be an alternation between melancholy and irritability (K. p. 1351: contradictory and alternating states). They can get angry as suddenly as NUX-V., VERAT. or STRAM. while they used to be so silent (It makes you think of the unexpected reaction you could get if you put salt in a fire).
- alternating symptoms: they can show very contradictory and alternating symptoms, mental and physical complaints can also alternate.
- hypochondriacal fear (K. p. 7: anxiety, hypochondriacal). They can get anxious about inanities, about a little spot on their skin and therefore come to the doctor. This symptom becomes strong when they are already deeply ill, and the fear may resemble PHOS. in such a state.

    D.d. ARS. and PHOS.: have this symptom too when they are superficially ill.
    NIT-AC.: are always hypochondriacal, even when healthy.

- fear of microbes and infection: they constantly want to wash their hands (NAT-M. may be added 2nd degree on p. 92: washing, always, her hands). With NAT-M., this symptom can be very strong: they can be so afraid of getting ill.

    D.d. SULPH.: Do this out of disgust (K. p. 37: disgust).
    NAT-M.: Do this in order not to get ill.
    SYPH.: Do this out of a kind of obsessive-compulsive neurosis.

- fear of heart disease: this can be so strong with NAT-M. that they are sure they have a heart disease, it can become an idée fixe. You can add NAT-M.1st degree in the rubric K. p. 45: fear, heart, disease of; beside KALI-ARS. 3rd degree and PHOS. 2nd degree.
- fear of narrow places and claustrophobia: In the opera, the cinema or in the bus, they are always near the exit. NAT-M. is very closed, if they see analogous situations round them, they get scared. You can add NAT-M. 1st degree in the rubric K. p. 46: fear, narrow place, in.
- fear of high places and dizziness if they are on high places. NAT-M. has this symptom very strongly (K. p. 100: vertigo, high places).
- fear in a crowd (K. p. 43: fear, crowd, in a).

- suicidal tendency: they can get suicidal tendencies which are difficult to distinguish from AURUM. They withdraw themselves and listen to melancholic music, this relieves their sadness (K. p. 62: loathing life).
  Contrary to AURUM., NAT-M. could be pleased with his depressive condition in a masochistic way.
- fear of a thunder storm (K. p. 47: fear, thunderstorm, of).

C. VERY DEEP MENTAL-EMOTIONAL PROBLEMS

If NAT-M. gets even more ill, we will see a mental and psychological picture that is the opposite of what we are used to.
This deeper situation is very difficult to diagnose. Mostly, this is only possible from information about the past (when the patient was very closed and serious), or by asking others.
In such a deep state, the patient can be very open, can speak like LACH., and can be without shame (resemble HYOS.).
E.g.: K. p. 79: shameless; shameless, bed, in: in case of a strong disturbance, they can start saying dirty words in bed, while making love. It is as if the beast in them comes up. They can use sadistic and masochistic language.
In a very deep disturbance, the patient can think a lot of death and become afraid of burglars (K. p. 1243: sleep, dream, robbers, and cannot sleep until the house is searched). Here, the d.d. with ARS. becomes difficult; they can both have the same symptoms:
- fear of diseases
- fear of microbes
- fear of burglars

6. THE EXTERNAL SIGNS OF NAT-M.

THE WHITE COLOUR

NAT-M. corresponds to salt. The colour of salt is white. This colour is seen everywhere on the outside of NAT-M.:

- white discharge from the eyes.
- white discharge from the nose (K. p. 333: nose, discharge, white, like white of eggs).
- white skin and white colour of the face.
- white-grey hair at a young age.
- white-coloured eruptions and white scales in the hair (K. p. 116: head, eruption, crusts and scabs, white).
- line of white eruptions on the hair line of the head.
- white aphthous ulcers in the mouth and on the gums.
- white vitiligo.
- white vaginal discharge (K. p. 723: genitalia, female, leucorrhoea, white).
- white spots on the nails.
- white-coloured vomit.
- white-coloured tongue with a red island in the centre (K. p. 402: mouth, discolouration, tongue, white patches, red insular with).
- white warts on the palms of the hands.

OTHER SIGNS

- Cracks in the lips and in the corners of the mouth (K. p. 357: face, cracked lips; cracked corners of mouth).
- Characteristic of NAT-M. is the herpes on the lips (K. p. face,

eruptions, herpes, mouth, around) as soon as they catch a cold or if they are emotionally disturbed.
- A horizontal line in the upper or lower eyelid.
- A small, slender neck with a small chest (K. p. 887: emaciation, cervical region; K. p. 829: emaciation, clavicles, about the).
- You sometimes see a serious general emaciation (K. p. 479: stomach, appetite, ravenous, emaciation with; K. p. 1358: emaciation, children).
- The genital hair sometimes fall out (K. p. 698: genitalia, hair, falling off; K. p. 718: genitalia, female, hair, falling out).

7. HOW WILL NAT-M. PRESENT THEM - SELVES IN THE CONSULTING-ROOM?

The idea of CLOSENESS and being INTROVERTED can be found everywhere and also during the consultation. Sometimes, NAT-M.-patients say they have an open character. Don't let yourself be fooled!! Ask them if they discuss their strictly personal problems with others. Sometimes, you can only know by asking others that they are silent, serious and withdrawn people.

Ask if the patient has personal problems or if he has had important setbacks or grief in his life. NAT-M. will give you a negative answer. Even when you feel that the patient is lying, don't insist! If you do, NAT-M. may shield even more and you won't get any more information. Instead of insisting, you should ask neutral questions, such as: about their eating habits, education, their childhood; sometimes, you may find an opening afterwards to go to more emotional questions.

If you, as a therapist, give a lot of love and affection to your NAT-M.-patient, they can seem very open. You might even think there is a PHOS.-patient in front of you. NAT-M. can be very open when they feel you are really fair to them.

The idea of closeness and being introverted can be found in the following symptoms:

- They sometimes think life is scaring, don't like this kind of life and dream of a society where nobody can hurt others.
- They have a fear of narrow places.
- They can be irritable and angry when you call their name loud in the waiting room.
- Very often, they don't even discuss their personal problems with their partner.
- When they are hurt, they keep everything inside them, don't want any company, don't talk about it with others and sometimes, nobody will see they are depressed.
- Sometimes, they say things like "Everybody has problems in the current society" or "The best solution for my problem is in myself".

8. GENERAL SYMPTOMS OF NAT-M.

- NAT-M. can be <u>chilly or warm blooded</u>: they are more warm blooded than NAT-C. and less warm blooded than NAT-S.

- They mostly <u>sleep on their left side</u>. They can dream that they are thirsty and looking for water the whole night (K. p. 1243: sleep, dreams, thirsty). They sometimes dream of burglars and can't sleep anymore until the whole house is searched (K. p. 1242: sleep, dreams, robbers, and cannot sleep until the house is searched). Children with this symptom don't want to sleep until their parents have searched the house.

- NAT-M. feels worse at the seaside (K. p. 1344: air, seashore), they can have a general aggravation. They may also say: "I feel well at the seaside, but the sun irritates me."

- NAT-M. can't bear the sun (K. p. 1404: sun, from exposure to). NAT-C. has this symptom even worse, that's why it is an important remedy for sunstroke.

- NAT-M.-patients know a periodicity in their symptoms (K. p. 1390: periodicity).

- NAT-M. feels better after perspiration.

- They can have problems after the use of quinine or after malaria, e.g. paralysis after malaria (K. p. 1397: quinine, abuse of).

- The worst time for NAT-M. is 10 a.m. (K. p. 1341: morning, 10 a.m.) or from 10 a.m. to 3 p.m. The headache and the fever are then worst. For asthma, worst time is 5 p.m. to 7 p.m.

- If they feel cold, the feeling of coldness will start in 1 finger and then extend to the whole body.

- They are dizzy on high places (K. p. 100: vertigo, high places), they can be dizzy while they are reading, and they have a tendency to fall to the left side in case of dizziness (K. p. 99: vertigo, fall, to left).

- The headache is mostly on the right side. During the headache, they may swear (may be added) and cry, as if they blame themselves. The headache is better with cold applications (K. p. 138: head, pain, cold applications amel.: NAT-M. may be added 3rd degree, next to ALOE.).

- In case of an inflammation of the eye caused by too strong light, by the sun on the snow or by welding: think of BELL. first, then of NAT-M.

- With diplopia, you must think of a serious neurologic affection, have the patient examined in time. One of the most important remedies for diplopia is NAT-M. (K. p. 277: vision, diplopia). With multiple sclerosis, we will often see this symptom.

According to Vassilis's experience, NAT-M. is the most important remedy for M.S.

- NAT-M. is mostly thirsty for icecold water in large quantities. Mostly, they have a dry mouth (K. p. 403: mouth, dryness, thirst, with; K. p. 529: stomach, thirst, large quantities, often for).

- NAT-M.-patients mostly have a good appetite and yet they are not fat. NAT-M.-children also eat a lot (d.d. IOD.).

- NAT-M. has a strong desire for the following things:
    - salt: NAT-M. is the strongest remedy for "desire salt" (K. p. 486: desires, salt).
    - fish (K. p. 485: desires, fish).
    - bitter (K. p. 484: desires, bitter drinks, bitter food).
    - pepper (K. p. 485: may be added 2nd degree).
    - oysters (K. p. 485: desires, oysters).
    - pasta (K. p. 485: desires, farinaceous food).
    - milk (K. p. 485: desires, milk); NAT-M. can also dislike milk.
    - bread (K. p. 484: desires, bread); NAT-M. can also dislike bread.

- NAT-M. dislikes the following things:
    - bread (K. p. 480: aversion, bread).
    - fat (K. p. 480: aversion, fat and rich food), this aversion is as strong as with PULS.
    - chicken (may be added 3rd degree).
    - slimy food (may be added 2nd degree next to CALC. and MED.).
    - fish (K. p. 482: aversion, fish).
    - salt (K. p. 482: aversion, salt food).
    - water (K. p. 482: aversion, water).

- NAT-M. likes the following things:
    - lemon: sometimes sprinkled with salt like VERAT. NAT-M. can be added 1st degree on K. p. 485: desires, lemon.
    - sometimes sour and vinegar like SEP.

- Concerning the genitalia, we see the following symptoms in NAT-M.:
    - pain during coitus (K. p. 734: pain, vagina, coition)
    - dry vagina (K. p. 717: dryness, vagina)
    - herpes on genitalia (K. p. 717: eruption, herpetic)
    - pubic hair falls out (K. p. 698: hair, falling off; K. p. 718: hair, falling out)
    - offensive perspiration (K. p. 701: odor, stinking)
    - involuntary childlessness (K. p. 744: sterility)

- In acute diseases, NAT-M. sometimes loses urine while coughing (K. p. 659: urination, involuntary, during cough).

- They can have restless legs in bed, like RHUS-T., SULPH. and MED. (K. p. 1188: restlessness, leg).

9. ACUTE SITUATIONS IN WHICH YOU HAVE TO THINK OF NAT-M.

- Lumbago and pain in the back by which the patient will lie down on the ground or on something very hard (K. p. 896: back, pain, lying, hard, on something, amel.).
- Headaches that start at 10 a.m. and that are better with cold applications. The headache is hammering.
- In a case of flu, they have shivers which start in 1 finger or toe and then extend to the whole body. The fever starts about 10 a.m. and mostly, there is herpes on the lips.
- In case of ailments from disappointed love by which the patient wants to be alone and weeps when nobody can see them. They mostly show herpes on the lips in such situations.

10. NAT-M. DURING PREGNANCY

- They mostly have constipation.
- They have a feeling as if the uterus is heavy, sometimes the feeling as if it wants to come out (K. p. 735: pain, bearing down, uterus).
- They often have anal loss of blood (K. p. 620: rectum, haemorrhoids, pregnancy, during).
- The eating habits may sometimes change a lot or become much stronger during the pregnancy: don't overlook this, it can be an important signal of the mother or her child.
  The desire for salt can increase. Sometimes a strong desire for fish, when they didn't eat fish before. Sometimes, the aversion to fat and slimy food becomes even stronger.
- During the pregnancy, NAT-M. can resemble SEP. very much. Then, you should still give NAT-M. if there were NAT-M.-signs before the pregnancy.

11. DIFFERENTIAL DIAGNOSIS OF NAT-M.

PHOSPHORUS (PHOS.)

- The constitutional information of NAT-M. can resemble PHOS. very much if NAT-M. appears more open or if PHOS. is not very open. If there are only physical problems, it can be very difficult to make a d.d. Then, you are forced to look at the smaller signs. If there are serious psychological problems, the choice will be easier.

- Similar information of NAT-M. and PHOS.:
    - hypochondriacal fears
    - afraid of thunder storms
    - sympathetic
    - desire for salt and fish (or aversion to fish)
    - very thirsty for large quantities of cold drinks

- When the choice between these 2 remedies is difficult, the following tips may help:
    - very thirsty for ice cold drinks is more PHOS.
    - serious fear of narrow places and serious dizziness on high places is mainly NAT-M.
    - very strong fear of thunderstorms is more PHOS.
    - very strong aversion to fat or slimy food is more NAT-M.
    - very strong desire for pasta is more NAT-M.
    - strong aversion to sweet is more PHOS.
    - very strong desire for ice cream will rather indicate PHOS.

- When there is confusion between the symptoms of NAT-M. and PHOS. and you find specific information for NAT-P., you will give NAT-P. of course.

    E.g.: - fear of thunderstorms
          - sympathetic
          - desire for salt
          - desire for fish: keynote of NAT-P.
          - desire for fried eggs: keynote of NAT-P.

SEPIA (SEP.)

- Similar information of NAT-M. and SEP.:
    - closed character
    - easily angry
    - depressed before the menses
    - aversion to coitus and pain during coitus

- When the choice between these two remedies is difficult, the following tips may help:
  - desire for vinegar and sweets is more SEP.
  - strong aversion to sex and continuous leucorrhoea is more SEP.
  - strong chilliness is more SEP.
  - strong desire for salt is more NAT-M.
  - strong aversion to fat is more NAT-M.
  - if the person can eat fat, better give SEP.
  - if the person can weep in company of others, or if the patient weeps during the interview, rather give SEP.
  - the feeling of a ball in the rectum is more indicated for SEP.
  - serious fear of heights and fear of narrow places is more NAT-M.
  - herpes round the lips will more indicate NAT-M.

- SEPIA-children are not so closed, they like to go to parties and like to dance. They easily provoke other children, and like to punish the others (even physically). NAT-M.-children on the contrary are never provocative and are very kind.

MEDORRHINUM (MED.)

- Similar information of NAT-M. and MED.:
  - closed character
  - losing weight
  - desire for salt and lemons (d.d. VERAT.)
  - aversion to slimy food (d.d. CALC.)
  - nailbiting

- When the choice is difficult, the following tips may help:
  - NAT-M. feels weak at night, MED. feels better at night.
  - MED. has a strong desire for salt, sweets, fat, sour and alcohol (NAT-M. mostly has an aversion to fat).
  - MED. has an amelioration of complaints at the seaside, where NAT-M. sometimes has an aggravation.
  - MED. mostly sleeps on the abdomen.

- If there is a swelling of the ankles, think of MED. immediately.
- MED. likes to eat ice cubes, or let them melt in the mouth.
- NAT-M. has more of a dislike for coitus than MED.
- MED. rather likes green, hard, unripe fruit.
- Immediately think of MED. when there is a fear of darkness and when there is a feeling as if someone is behind them or in the same room (the feeling of a presence).

PULSATILLA (PULS.)

- Similar information of NAT-M. AND PULS.:
  - aversion to fat (fat of meat, chicken or bacon)
  - sensitive
  - aggravation in the sun or headache caused by the sun
  - depressed before or during the menses

- When the choice between NAT-M. and PULS. is difficult, the following tips may help:
  - thirstlessness: rather give PULS.
  - PULS. will also weep in company of others
  - NAT-M. usually has constipation during the menses

12. ANTIDOTES FOR NAT-M.

MENTHOL, even the odor of it may antidote NAT-M. The prepacked tissues to clean the fingers contain menthol. The dentist will use them sometimes.

13. COMPLEMENTARY REMEDIES

- **IGNATIA**
- **SEPIA**
- **ARGENTUM NITRICUM**

LYC. will follow well after NAT-M.

NATRUM SULPHURICUM : ESSENCE

It is the second most frequent of the NATRUMs after NAT-M.
It is the least sensitive of all NATRUMs. NAT-S. is more materialistic, more earthly (like GRAPH. or BRY.). NAT-S. is the remedy for BUSINESSMEN with successful jobs, a lot of money, having a nice career.

1. NAT-S. ON THE MENTAL-EMOTIONAL LEVEL

THE NAT-S.-CHILD

They often suffer from ASTHMA at a young age (K. p. 764: respiration, asthmatic, children; K. p. 768: respiration, difficult, children). Possibly, the parents had gonorrhoea or condylomata which had been treated allopathicly. The asthma begins at the age of 4 or 5 and will disappear about the age of 15 or by allopathic treatment or by emotional suppression.

THE NAT-S.-ADOLESCENT

Their body is weakened by the asthma and they are constantly confronted with their limits on the physical plane. They try very hard to be the best at school, in spite of their handicap. They study very much but aren't always the top of the class like AURUM. They continuously compare themselves with those who are better than them. They thus become competitive minded and develop a REVENGEFULNESS towards their classmates who achieve better results. NAT-S. has this revengefulness in common with AURUM. These are the two remedies that can have the greatest SUICIDAL TENDENCIES.

The NAT-S.-adolescent tries to compensate for his physical weakness by working more systematically (NAT-S. is the remedy that can work most systematically). In addition, they have a strong SENSE OF DUTY and a strong SENSE OF RESPONSIBILITY (like AURUM).

THE NAT-S.-ADULT

- The combination of working systematically, a strong sense of duty and a strong sense of responsibility makes them a prototype of the successful businesman (more men than women). They have a good job, a lot of money, several cars, possess properties or factories, have often a lot of power. They work very hard, suppress everything that has nothing to do with their work. They are very often surrounded by people who depend on them and with whom they have a close bond. NAT-S.-patients like people who depend on them and people who need them. They for their part give a lot to them.

- NAT-S. remains always REVENGEFUL when they see someone else who is also trying to be the best. NAT-S. is the great PLANNER. They are very systematic and plan everything for the future. They will make sure their daughter will have a house, their son will get a good business and their wife will have enough money in her account.

- NAT-S. doesn't have a good emotional relationship with the people surrounding them. The only things that count for them are their job and their success. The only persons they have a good relationship with are their wife and children. Yet, they like the bond with the people surrounding them. With the therapist too, there is no real close bond. NAT-S. can talk in a very professional, cool and objective way about their physical problems. Sometimes, as a therapist you may feel a bit inferior towards those people.

- NAT-S. is a PEACEMAKER. They can't stand quarrels. They will always try to mediate when people are having arguments.

- NAT-S. is not choosy while looking for a partner. They mostly have little sexual experience because the only thing that matters to them is their work. If however, they find a partner, they will be besotted with love and they will worship their partner. They can only see the positive side of the partner and are blind to their shortcomings. Even if the partner is not fair, or his wife were to have a relationship with other men, they won't believe this or don't want to hear it. NAT-S. can't stand others speaking badly of their partner. They are pleased as long as the partner stays with them. If the partner leaves them, they will suddenly get physically ill (not psychologically): they can get their asthma back or develop an ulcer. It is a real ulcer or real asthma (don't be mistaken with tightness of the chest in IGN. after grief).

- In general, NAT-S. is not irritable and not easily angry. The only exception to this rule is when you insult or accuse their partner (with or without good reason).

- NAT-S. likes soft music. Music makes them feel better for a while (the idea of romanticism). So, you can see a very serious successful businessman in a bar crying quietly with faint light and beautiful music (K. p. 94: weeping, music, from).

- NAT-S. will feel better after stool when they are depressed or melancholic. They sometimes say the best time of the day is the morning. Ask then if it is not after the stool in the morning (K. p. 11: cheerful, stools, after).

NAT-S. HAS STRONG SUICIDAL TENDENCIES

NAT-S. feels psychologically well as long as everything goes well. They can be tired however because of the pressure of the responsibility and the burden of work and may get into psychologically difficult situations: at that moment, they will have suicidal tendencies (K. p. 85: suicidal disposition). However, so many people depend on them that they can't commit suicide immediately because of the others. They will plan everything: first, their family must be safe. Their wife shan't lack anything. The future of their children must be safe and their family must be able to do without them. Then, they'll plan how to commit suicide. As long as there is any indication that their family isn't put out of harm's way, they will not proceed to the act (K. p. 63: loathing, life, must restrain herself to prevent doing herself injury). If everything is going as planned and they commit suicide, NAT-S. will chose death by HANGING (K. p. 85: suicidal disposition, hanging, by). (AURUM would rather jump from a high place: the jump to freedom).

2. NAT-S. ON THE PHYSICAL LEVEL

ASTHMA

- This is the most important complaint for NAT-S.
- It can be seen in children whose parents had gonorrhoea or condylomata (K. p. 670: urethra, discharge, gonorrhoeal; K. p. 693: genitalia, condylomata).
- The expectoration is green-yellow and the tongue is coloured green to grey (K. p. 816: expectoration, greenish; K. p. 401: mouth, discolouration, tongue, green; discolouration, tongue, greenish, gray).

- They have a sensation as if the thorax is empty or that it will break: that's why they always hold their chest in an attack of asthma (K. p. 792: cough, hands, must hold chest with both, while).
- The asthma is aggravated by wet or foggy weather: warm, wet weather is worst (K. p. 1413: warm wet weather agg.; K. p. 772: respiration, difficult, wet weather).
- The asthma is worst about 4 or 5 a.m. (K. p. 764: respiration, asthmatic, midnight, after, 4 to 5 a.m.).
- Think of it in asthma patients with a history of gonorrhoea or condylomata. Even if the person had the gonorrhoea treated allopathicly and afterwards got condylomata.

HEADACHE

- Most characteristic is the photophobia during the headache (K. p. 262: eye, photophobia, headache, during).
- There is a bitter taste in the mouth and they suffer from indigestion during the headache.
- They vomit pure bile during the headache (K. p. 535: stomach, vomiting, bile, headache, with): this symptom is again characteristic of NAT-S.
- The combination of liver problems and headache is typical of NAT-S. The patient says he has a headache when his liver or gall bladder don't function very well or that he vomits because the headache is working on his gall-bladder. (In the chinese philosophy, the liver is the organ that represents planning).
- The headache is better by pressure and in open air.
- Headaches after skull or brain trauma (K. p. 141: head, pain, injuries, mechanical, after).

COLITIS

- The diarrhœa is worst in the morning after rising (K. p. 609: rectum, diarrhœa, morning, rising, after): it is a sputtering stool (K. p. 642: stool, sputtering) with a lot of offensive flatus.
- The diarrhœa is aggravated by eating green vegetables (K. p. 615: rectum, diarrhœa, vegetables, after) and by pasta (K. p. 613: rectum, diarrhœa, food, farinaceous, after).

SKULL INJURIES

- NAT-S. is the most important remedy for injuries of the head (K. p. 128: head, injuries of the head, after).
- Characteristic of NAT-S. is the change of personality or character after an accident.
  In fact, you have to think of it after trauma of whatever part of the body (even the neck), if there has been a change in the patient's personality.
  It is possible that the patient will be depressed after the accident (K. p. 77: sadness, injuries of the head, from), irritable, get suicidal tendencies, go mad (K. p. 56: insanity, injuries to the head, from; K. p. 15: confusion, injury to head, after) and even will have to be treated in a psychiatric hospital with psychopharmacologic drugs. In the repertory, you can create a new rubric: mental symptoms from injuries = NAT-S. 3rd degree.
- Epilepsy after an accident or after a skull trauma (K. p. 1354: convulsions, injuries, from). If there was a subdural haematoma, even if it has been drained, give ARN. first, before NAT-S.

OTHER INFORMATION

- NAT-S. can have jaundice after anger or vexation (K. p. 1307: skin, discoloration, yellow, jaundice, vexation). Very often, the liver or gall-bladder will be affected (K. p. 553: abdomen, inflammation, liver, chronic; K. p. 568: abdomen, pain, liver, colic, gall stones).
- With genital condylomata or genital warts, you have to think of NAT-S. (K. p. 693: genitalia, condylomata; K. p. 715: genitalia, female, condylomata).
- In case of intestinal cancer, but especially with sigmoid cancer, you have to think of NAT-S. If there is a peculiar change in the stool habits with serious constipation or constipation that alternates with diarrhœa, have the patient examined and think of cancer. In the rubric on K. p. 606: rectum, cancer: you can add NAT-S.

D.d. ALUM. : has to get out the stool with his fingers.
      NIT-AC.: miserable persons with an enormeous fear of cancer.
      SEP.: feels a ball in the rectum.

3. GENERAL INFORMATION OF NAT-S.

TEMPERATURE SENSITIVINESS

NAT-S. is mostly warm blooded. They like to uncover their feet because the soles of the feet are hot (K. p. 1012: heat, foot, evening). The top of their head is warm too, like SULPH. Sometimes however, their whole back is cold (K. p. 884: back, coldness).
NAT-S. has most problems in warm, wet weather (K. p. 143: warm, wet weather, agg.).

EATING HABITS

NAT-S. is <u>aggravated by eating green vegetables</u> (K. p. 1364: food, vegetables, green, agg.), by pasta (K. p. 1363: food, farinaceous food agg.) and by milk. They have an aversion to bread (K. p. 480: aversion, bread) and sometimes to meat. They like food that was preserved in salt. They are thirsty and like cold drinks (K. p. 484: desires, cold drinks) with ice cubes in it.

STOOL AMELIORATES ALL COMPLAINTS

With NAT-S., every symptom or every complaint can disappear after stool. The patient can also feel better after stool, both mentally and psychologically (K. p. 11: cheerful, after stool).

4. COMPLEMENTARY REMEDIES TO NAT-S.

The most important <u>complementary remedy</u> of NAT-S. is <u>MEDORRHINUM</u> (they are also complementary in the other way).

5. DIFFERENTIAL DIAGNOSIS WITH NAT-S.

AURUM METALLICUM (AUR.)

Here, d.d. is very difficult. Mostly, AUR. suffers a lot in silence. You can sometimes see that they are suffering, but they will never speak about their bad situation and about their suicidal tendencies.

NAT-S. doesn't suffer as much as AUR. NAT-S. won't commit suicide so easily because of their family and children. If NAT-S. has provided all material things for their family, they are easy and calm. NAT-S. will sooner talk about their suicidal tendencies and will say that they would commit suicide if they didn't have children. If they lost their family, you can be sure they would do it.

SULPHUR (SULPH.)

There is a lot of identical information between SULPH. and NAT-S. Give NAT-S. if you see the characteristic headache or asthma of NAT-S. (mentioned above).

THUJA (THUJ.)

NAT-S. can be easily confused with THUJA because of the condylomata.

If you have a patient who is suspicious, who gives you the feeling that he doesn't appreciate you very much, who has condylomata and who perspires with a peculiar sweet odor, think of THUJA.

MEDORRHINUM (MED.)

If the patient shows condylomata, wants to uncover his feet, desires fat and salt, likes sour things and has swollen ankles, give MED.

CHINA OFFICINALIS (CHIN.)

- CHINA is also aggravated by wet and damp weather. Here, the appetite is bad (K. p. 479: stomach, appetite, wanting, foggy weather, in).
- CHINA has also stomach troubles with possible colitis: there is especially flatulence and swelling of the abdomen, especially if there are gall-bladder problems (as in NAT-S.).
- CHINA has a strong desire for sweets (K. p. 486: stomach, desires, sweets).

CHELIDONIUM MAJUS (CHEL.)

- With CHEL., we also find affections of liver and gall-bladder.
- If they have a headache because of the liver or gall-bladder, it will mostly be situated above the right eye (K. p. 159: head, pain, forehead, eyes, above right).
- Characteristic of CHEL. is also the pain in the right hypochondrium which extends to the right shoulder blade (K. p. 564: abdomen, pain, hypochondria, extending to scapula).
- Characteristic is also the pain which goes through the body like a knife that is stabbed in the body from one side to the other (K. p. 561: abdomen, pain, extending across; extending transversally).

REMEDIES AND THEIR CHARACTERISTIC SYMPTOMS IN COMMON COLDS

EUPATORIUM PERFOLIATUM (EUP-PER)

- These patients show a suddenly appearing flu syndrome. Sometimes, it is an epidemic.
- Mostly, the fever isn't very high and there is little cough.
- The main complaint is <u>pain in all bones and joints.</u>
  The pain is wandering around in the body. Characteristic is also the feeling <u>as if they were beaten.</u> (Pain sore, bruised: K. p. 1125, 1126 and next.)
  Usually, the pain is situated in the long bones.
- They are very <u>thirsty for cold drinks</u> (K. p. 484: desire cold drinks). They desire ice cream (K. p. 485).
- They are restless and anxious.
- <u>Internally, they are very warm, but externally, they feel cold.</u> They have a warm feeling on the top of their head.
- They have a pulsating headache, aggravated by lying down.
- The picture makes you think of PHOS., because of the strong desire for cold drinks and ice cream, of ARS. while they are anxious and restless and sometimes of BRY. or RHUS-T.

FERRUM PHOSPHORICUM (FERR-P)

- These patients have a very fast rising fever. The symptoms of the disease look like GELS.
- You should think of it when there is a continuous fever without any other symptom (in such a case, always think of the possibility of pneumonia!).
  If, however, there is a continuous fever without any other symptom and the patient is very weak and exhausted (prostration), you have to think of KALI-P.

CAUSTICUM (CAUST.)

What are the characteristics of CAUST. in case of an acute common cold?

- Loss of urine during cough and laughing
  Hierarchy of remedies in the rubric "Urination involuntary during cough" (K. p. 659) :
  1. CAUST.   2. SEP.   3. PULS.   4. NAT-M.   5. SQUILL.
  6. APIS.
- In an acute situation, they are always chilly.
- They are better in damp or rainy weather (Wet weather amel.: rubric added by Vithoulkas). If the patient says that wet weather ameliorates his hay fever or his allergy or rheumatic pains, think first of all of CAUST.
- They have dryness in throat or a sore throat with the feeling that there is mucus in the trachea (K. p. 457: throat, mucus, swallow, which must). They try to hawk it up, but in vain (K. p. 453: throat, hawk, disposition to, ineffectual; K. p. 785: cough, deep enough, sensation as though he could not cough, to start mucus).
- Cough is ameliorated by cold drinks (K. p. 784: cough, cold drinks amel.; d.d. CUPRUM METALLICUM).
- In case of whooping cough, they can 't stop their cough.
  The face becomes blue with coughing (K. p. 358: face, discoloration bluish, cough, during). Drinking something cold ameliorates the cough.

(Cough, ameliorated by warm drinks are other remedies: K. p. 810: cough, warm fluids amel.)
- In an acute disease, they sometimes have the feeling that something very bad will happen to them (K. p. 45: fear, happen, something will; d.d. PHOS.).
- Sometimes, they have a feeling as if drops of cold water run down the back. If you see this symptom and the patient is chilly, think of CAUST.; if the patient is warm blooded, think of PULS. (LYC. doesn't show this symptom very much). You should add CAUST. at K. p. 885: back, coldness, extending down back, as if cold water poured down the.
- They can be very thirsty, but they mostly have an aversion to water (K. p. 482: aversion water), and a desire for beer (K. p. 484: desires beer).
- In an acute disease, they can be hungry, and from the moment they sit down to the table and see food, the hunger disappears and they can't get any food down (K. p. 478: appetite increased, vanishing at sight of food; idem for KALI-C.).

  d.d. LYC.: they begin to eat, but immediately feel such a fullness in the abdomen that they can't eat any more (K. p. 476: appetite, easy satiety).

- In case of facial paralysis (K. p. 390: paralysis, facial) you must think of ACON. the first day. From the 3rd or 4th day, think of CAUST.
- Loss of voice or hoarseness (K. p. 759: voice, hoarseness, coryza, during), especially a sudden loss of voice during a flu must make you think of CAUST.
- CAUST. is aggravated in the morning, particularly the feeling of mucus in throat and trachea is worst then. When they rise in the morning, they try hard to get out some mucus, and they feel better if they succeed.

HEPAR SULPHURIS (HEP.)

- Their sore throat is ameliorated by warm drinks (K. p. 459: throat, pain, warm drinks amel.) and warm applications (K. p. 459: throat, pain, warmth in general amel.).
- They have a deep dry cough like a dog who barks (K. p. 782: cough, barking). Their coughing makes them short of breath and they have a sensation of suffocation in the throat.
- In an acute situation, they are extremely chilly (more than ARS.). They want a lot of blankets on themselves or they are dressed with several layers of clothes one on top of another (like an onion).
- In a chronic situation, HEP. is also chilly. Don't give HEP. if someone is warm blooded.
- They start to sneeze or to cough from the least uncovering, even by uncovering one hand (K. p. 809: cough, uncovering hands).
- Their cough is aggravated by:
    - the least uncovering (K. p. 809: cough, uncovering agg.)
    - cold, open air or a draft of air (K. p. 781: cough, air cold)
    - cold drinks (K. p. 784: cough, cold drinks)
    - talking (K. p. 807: cough, talking)
    - before midnight

SPONGIA TOSTA (SPONG.)

- This is not a deep working remedy, but it is very useful with acute common colds and cough.
- In an acute disease, there is a cough which is ameliorated by eating sweets (K. p. 790: cough, eating amel.) or by warm drinks (K. p. 786: cough, drinking amel.; K. p. 810: cough, warm fluids amel.).
- In case of a chronic cough, they often have a bottle of water or some sweets with them. When coughing, they take a sweet or sip and say: "This is my best remedy, it makes the cough stop right away."

RUMEX CRISPUS (RUMEX.)

- They have a cough with white expectoration which becomes yellow and thick and is difficult to bring up.
  The <u>cough is aggravated by every change of temperature</u> (K. p. 810: cough, warm room, going from, to cold air, or vice versa, agg.; d.d. PHOS.).
- A change of temperature can also make them sneeze.
- They have a sore throat and are hoarse (because of the mucus).
- There is an aggravation of cough at 11 p.m. (K. p. 781: cough, night, 11 p.m.), even in their sleep (d.d. LACH. cough at that time only when they are asleep, not if they are awake).

GELSEMIUM (GELS.)

- During an acute disease, their <u>eyelids are very heavy</u> and fall down (K. p. 241: eye, heaviness lids). They wish they had something to keep them open.
- They easily <u>tremble from weakness</u> (K. p. 1408: trembling externally); that's why they don't want any company and don't want to be disturbed (K. p. 37: disturbed, aversion to being).

    <u>d.d. Company aversion to</u> (K. p. 12)

-<u>GELS.</u>:	they are too weak, lose too much energy if they have company
-<u>NAT-M.</u>:	introverted, and if they talk, they will have persistant thoughts afterwards.
-<u>NUX-V.</u>:	in company, there can be a confrontation with others and then, they become irritable.
-<u>BAR-C.</u>:	they are childish and say that everybody is laughing at them.

- In an acute disease, GELS. is <u>thirstless</u> (K. p. 530: stomach, thirstless, heat, during; d.d. BRY.). If very thirsty, you'd better not give them GELS.

- They perspire and are wet all over the body. Their clothes stick to the body; nevertheless, they are thirstless.
- They have an empty feeling in their chest. Also the feeling that their heart will stop, which makes them walk around to lose this feeling (K. p.824: chest, cease, fears, unless constantly on the move, the heart will cease: K. p. 45 fear, heart will cease to beat unless constantly on the move; K. p. 44 fear of death).

RHUS-TOXICODENDRON (RHUS-T.)

- They are restless, can't sit still or lie down very long, and have to walk around. They are restless in their sleep, have to get up at times.
- They have restless feet (K. p. 1188: restlessness feet), they twist their feet around as if they want to stretch the ankle-joints. So, they can twist or stretch every joint (even the neck). Sometimes, they put a weight on their feet to do so: e.g. they let a child sit on their feet and then move their feet.
- During an acute disease, they sometimes can't stop thinking, always the same idea is running through their head (like theorizing of CANN-I.). They enjoy these persistent thoughts. (K. p. 87: thoughts, persistent).

  d.d. NAT-M. : they are always thinking about bad things, and worrying.
  NAT-C. : they are masochistic, won't stop worrying.

- They dream and have the feeling that they work hard in their dream (K. p. 1237: sleep, dreams, business of), or e.g. walk fast against the wind.
- In case of a RHUS-T. cold in the nose, we will see a nose obstruction in alternating sides, depending on the side they are lying on: lying on the left side gives an obstruction of the left nostril, on the right side one of the right nostril.
  (to add in the repertory K. p. 341: obstruction, nose, side, lying on: RHUS-T.)

BARYTA MURIATICA (BAR–M.)

- They have an earache which is ameliorated by cold drinks.
  (K. p. 304: ear, pain, cold drinks amel.).
- Mostly, there is a sore throat with swollen or enlarged tonsils.
  (K. p. 451: enlargement of tonsils; K. p. 469: swelling, tonsils).
- They mostly have a nasal obstruction.
- They are chilly, get worse from cold drinks and nevertheless like
  cold drinks.
- All the cervical glands and the glands around the neck are swollen
  (K. p. 948: back, swelling, glands of nape).

SULPHUR (SULPH.)

What are the characteristics of SULPH. in an acute common cold?

- In an acute disease, 90 % are warm blooded and only 10 % chilly.
- They are very thirsty (K. p. 529: thirst, large quantities for).
- They have a burning sensation in the eyes. They have a feeling as
  if there is sand in their eyes (K. p. 258: eye, pain, sand, as from):
  this is the keynote of SULPH. in an acute disease. They have
  discharge from the eyes which is yellow, thick and even
  offensive. They continuously try to get the sand out of their eyes.
  (If the eye trouble disappears by cold applications, think first of
  PULS.)
- In an acute disease, you will very often find that they have
  burning hot feet which they want to uncover (K. p. 1013: heat
  foot, burning, uncovers them).
  SULPH.'s whole foot is hot, while LYC. only has hot soles.
  Even if SULPH. is chilly, they will uncover their feet in an acute
  disease.
- In the morning, the eyes are easily stuck up by a thick yellow
  discharge (K. p. 235: eye, agglutinated, morning). We find this
  symptom even in hay fever.
- They perspire, and their perspiration is offensive.

- In case of a common cold, they very often have a frontal headache which is ameliorated by cold applications (K. p. 156: head, pain, forehead, cold applications amel.)(you can be sure of SULPH. if they also uncover their feet).
- They mostly have very red lips in an acute disease (K. p. 363: face, discoloration, red lips).
- The cough is worst at night.
- Very often, the common cold goes together with offensive diarrhoea, if you absolutely don't have any other information, you could think of SULPH.

PULSATILLA NIGRICANS (PULS.)

What are the characteristics of PULS. in an acute common cold?

- In an acute situation, they weep easily (K. p. 93: weeping, heat, during the).
  Weep most in an acute situation: PULS.
  Weep chronically more than any other remedy: SEP.
- They are thirstless (K. p. 530: thirstless).
- The colour of the discharge from the nose is not important. PULS. has all the colours of the rainbow.
- They have a dry cough which is aggravated in every circumstance by lying down (even during the daytime).
  (K. p. 789: Cough, dry, lying, while: is 90 % PULS., 7 % SPONG. and 2 % HYOS).
  Even in case of a chronic problem or asthma: if their cough is dry while lying down, think of PULS. Coughing in bed only at night makes you think of other remedies.
- They have a cough that can be dry at night and loose in the morning (K. p. 787: cough, dry, night, loose by day).
- The cough is always aggravated by warmth, by the sun as well as a warm place, a fire or warm drinks (K. p. 793: cough, heated, on becoming; K. p. 810: cough, warm, on becoming; K. p. 810: cough, warm room; cough, warm food).

- They cough by exertion or walking fast (K. p. 790: cough, exertion, violent; K. p. 810 cough, walking fast).
- They lose urine if they cough (K. p. 659: urination, involuntary, cough, during) (with a chilly person, first think of CAUST.).
- They get a cold easily if they get wet (K. p. 1421: wet, getting, feet; wet, getting, head; d.d. RHUSTOX, CAUST., DULC., RAN-B.).
- In an acute disease, they can have a strong desire for lemonade (K. p. 485: desire lemonade; d.d. BELL.).
- The cough gets worse if they get warm in bed (K. p. 782: cough, bed, warm, on becoming in, agg or excites). If the cough comes up only after a few hours in bed, rather think of SULPH.

KALI-BICHROMICUM (KALI-BI.)

- The main problem is mostly situated in the nose, with nasal obstruction or sinusitis, together with yellow discharge from nose looking like cheese spread (K. p. 332: nose, discharge, viscid, tough).
- The nose obstruction often goes together with a headache and pain on the base of the nose (K. p. 344: nose, pain, root).
- The worst hours for KALI-BI., like for all KALI's, are between 2 and 4 a.m. (K. p. 1343: night 2 a.m.).
- Sometimes, they wheeze, which is caused by a thick discharge coming down from the throat to the trachea.

SEPIA (SEP.)

- Not many characteristic symptoms in case of common cold.
- With SEP., the expectoration causes nausea or vomiting. (K. p. 533: vomiting, hawking up mucus, when).

ANTIMONIUM TARTARICUM (ANT-T.)

- Think of ANT-T. with seriously ill patients having a very hard cough: <u>you get the impression that the patient must hawk up masses of mucus but nothing comes up</u> (K. p. 807: cough rattling).

ARNICA MONTANA (ARN.)

- ARN. is well known as a remedy for INJURIES. The keynote of ARN. is the haematoma (external or internal).
- In acute common colds, ARN. is more difficult to find, and d.d. with SULPH. is not easy.
- In case of an acute disease, ARN. mostly shows a symptom of <u>eructations smelling like spoiled eggs</u> (K. p. 493: eructation, eggs, spoiled like). However, SULPH. has more this symptom than ARN.
- They can also be flatulent with flatus smelling like spoiled eggs (K. p. 618: flatus offensive, spoiled eggs).
- They have the feeling that their <u>bed is much too hard</u>, as if the mattress is full of stones or their pillow too hard, which makes them change their position (K. p. 1365: hard bed, sensation of; d.d. RHUST.).
- They are irritable when you examine them, they don't like to be touched (K. p. 43: fear approaching him , of others, lest he be touched; d.d. BRY.).
- Vassilis never saw the symptom of sending the doctor away.
  (K. p. 59: irritability, sends the doctor home, says he is not ill)

WYETHIA HELENOIDES (WYE.)

- Is best known as a remedy for hay fever (see later).
- Their headache has something in common with GLON.: they have the feeling that all their blood raises to the head.
- They have a tendency to clear their throat or to cough continuously.
- They have an <u>itching sensation deep in their throat or on the palate</u> and they try to scratch it with their tongue (K. p. 454: throat, itching).

REMEDIES AND THEIR CHARACTERISTIC SYMPTOMS IN TONSILLITIS

NO. 1 MERCURIUS IODATUS FLAVUS (MERC-I-F)

- If there are no constitutional symptoms and if the only complaint is an acute right-sided tonsillitis, you have a chance of 60 % that MERC-I-F. will help the patient (more than BELL. and LYC.). (K. p. 453: throat, inflammation, right; K. p. 458: throat, pain, right; K. p. 469: swelling, tonsils, right)

NO. 2 MERCURIUS IODATUS RUBER (MERC-I-R.)

- In an acute left tonsillitis, MERC-I-R. mostly works better than LACH. (unless you need LACH. constitutionally) (K. p. 453: throat, inflammation, left; K. p. 469: swelling, tonsils, left).
- Mostly, the patient can't swallow very well.
- MERC-I-F. occurs more often and works better than MERC-I-R.

NO. 3   MERCURIUS SOLUBILIS (MERC.)

- In case of tonsillitis accompanied by <u>salivation at night during sleep</u> (K. p. 418: salivation, night; salivation, sleep, during).

- With MERC., you will always find the following symptoms:
  - They have offensive breath (K. p. 409: mouth, odor, offensive).
  - There is perspiration, especially at night (K. p. 1294: perspiration, night, lasting all night without relief).
  - They are very sensitive to cold and heat.
  - They want to drink cold water (K. p. 484: desires cold drinks).

- If, after MERC-I-F., the sore throat of a patient with acute right tonsillitis is better after 2 days on the right side and gets worse on the left side and the patient feels generally better, you should give MERC. SOL. to complete the cure.
- MERC. is used more successfully in acute tonsillitis than LYC. or LACH. (K. p. 454: inflammation, tonsils).

LACHESIS (LACH.)

- Acute <u>left tonsillitis</u> which gets better by cold drinks (d.d. APIS.) (K. p. 458: throat, pain, left; throat, pain, cold drinks amel.).
- If the pain in the throat starts on the left side and afterwards extends to the right side (K 1401: side, left then right).
- Be careful with LACH.: this is a deep working constitutional remedy by which you easily get a proving. By rapidly repeating LACH., you can get complicated cases.

LYCOPODIUM (LYC.)

- Acute right tonsillitis (K. p. 458: throat, pain, right).
- If the pain starts on the right side and changes to the left side (K 1401: side, right then left).
- Generally prefer warm drinks (K. p. 486: desire warm drinks).
- However, in case of an acute disease, they prefer cold drinks according to Vassilis (K. p. 458: throat, pain, cold drinks amel).

HEPAR SULPHURIS (HEP.)

- HEP. is very, very chilly, especially in acute diseases.
- The tonsillitis is ameliorated by warm drinks (K. p. 459: throat, pain, warm drinks amel).
- HEP. is often used for pharyngitis, especially when they have a feeling as if there is a fish bone in their throat (K. p. 464: throat pain, splinter, as from a).
- HEP. can also be used for an abscess behind the tonsil, by which the throat is completely swollen on one side (if so, incision is mostly necessary) (K. p. 467: suppuration tonsils).

BARYTA MURIATICA (BAR-M.)

- They have enormously swollen tonsils (K. p. 469: swelling tonsils).
- Very often, they have swelling of glands at other places too, with hard and painful glands (K. p. 474: external, throat, swelling cervical glands; swelling cervical glands, hard).
- They mostly can't hear very well because of obstruction of the Eustachian tube.
- Rather use BAR-M. than BAR-C. in case of an acute disease, as BAR-C. is used more constitutionally. You may think of BAR-C. if the patient can't swallow anymore (K. p. 468: throat, swallowing difficult, solids).

NITRICUM ACIDUM (NIT-AC.)

- They have <u>offensive breath</u>, without salivation (K. p. 409: mouth, odor, cadaverous).
- They have also <u>pain as if there is a fish bone in the throat</u>. (K. p. 464: throat, pain, splinter, as from a).
- Mostly, they also have other stinging pains (K. p. 1385: pain, splinter, sensation of) and offensive perspiration on several places (K. p. 1299: perspiration, odor, urine like, horses).

APIS MELLIFICA (APIS.)

- Here, we have serious swellings which look as if they will burst.
- The <u>uvula is very swollen</u> as if it would burst (K. p. 469: throat swelling uvula).
- The <u>tonsils are very swollen</u> and give the impression that they will explode.
- Complaints are ameliorated by drinking cold (K. p. 458: throat, pain, cold drinks amel).

BELLADONNA (BELL.)

- In 80 % of the cases, the complaint is on the <u>right</u> side, exceptionally left (K. p. 1400: side, symptom on one side, right).
- Necessarily, you will find a <u>hot head and cold extremities</u>. (K. p. 122: head, heat, coldness of extremities, with).
- A BELL. sore throat can't bear the slightest touch (K. p. 1407: touch, slight, agg.).
- Mostly, you will find a strong photophobia (K. p. 262: eye, photophobia, chill, during).
- In an acute situation, BELL. likes sour drinks such as lemonade (K. p. 485: desires lemonade).

-   When repeating BELL., be careful for proving such as strong photophobia or headache with cold extremities.

With <u>**tonsillitis,**</u> **as always in homœopathy, pay attention to priority symptoms and to the most striking, strongest symptoms.**

E.g.: - offensive breath: in hierarchical order:
            1st = MERC.,
            2nd = NIT-AC.
            3rd = HEP.

  - a lot of salivation during sleep: first of all MERC.

    - feeling as if a fish bone in the throat: HEP. as well as NIT-AC.:
        > if the patient is extremely chilly, HEP. should score higher,
        > if the breathing is offensive and the patient stinks, rather prefer NIT-AC.

REMEDIES AND THEIR CHARACTERISTIC SYMPTOMS IN WHOOPING COUGH AND SEVERE COUGH

NO. 1   BELLADONNA (BELL.)

- They have a <u>violent cough which is almost suffocating</u> (K. p. 800: cough persistent).
- They are very afraid that they will suffocate and die. The child wants to be with his mother and wants to feel her (d.d. ARS. - PHOS.).
- The cough is worse at night (K. p. 805: cough spasmodic night).
- They have a <u>warm head with cold extremities</u> (K. p. 122: head, heat, coldness of extremities, with). With the fits of coughing, the face is red and warm, it radiates warmth.
- They have sudden attacks of violent and suffocating coughing with fear.
- Sometimes, the cough goes together with sneezing (K. p. 804: cough, sneezing, ends in), sometimes it is accompanied by strong photophobia.

NR. 2 CUPRUM METALLICUM (CUPR.)

- The cough stops when they drink something cold (K. p. 784: cough, cold drinks amel.).
- The cough comes up in fits. Face and lips may discolor blue by the spastic fits of coughing.
- The cough may be accompanied by cramps.

NR. 3 DROSERA (DROS.)

- They have frequent paroxysmal fits of coughing succeeding so fast that the child has the feeling as if he has no time to breathe (K. p. 800: cough, paroxysmal, attacks follow one another quickly).
- Most attacks are after midnight (K. p. 799: cough paroxysmal, night, midnight, after). D.d. KALI'S. (K. p. 799: cough, paroxysmal, night, midnight, after, 2 a.m.).
- Between the attacks, the child is restless and wants to walk around (d.d. ARS.).
- Characteristic of DROS. is the epistaxis with whooping cough or ordinary cough (K. p. 337: nose epistaxis cough with; epistaxis, cough with, whooping cough).
- While coughing, the patient must hold his abdomen or chest because of the pain (K. p. 792: cough, hands, must hold chest with both, while; holding pit of stomach amel.).
- In case of whooping cough, the patient has a fever which starts in the morning and lasts until night. In the day, the patient does not perspire, at night there is a warm perspitation on face, abdomen and stomach.

NR. 4   CAUSTICUM (CAUST.)

- See: common colds.
- The cough is ameliorated by drinking something cold.
- Mostly, there is loss of urine while coughing.

NR. 5   COCCUS CACTI (COC–C.)

- They have paroxysmal fits of coughing while the face colours blue.
- The expectoration is sticky and stringy (K. p. 820: expectoration, viscid).
- Worst time is before midnight at 11.30 p.m. (K. p. 799: cough, paroxysmal, night, midnight before, 11.30 p.m.).

NR. 6   IPECACUANHA (IP.)

- Here, it is necessary that the patient vomits while coughing.
  (K. p. 532: stomach, vomiting, coughing on)
- The tongue is clean, in spite of the vomiting.
- Never give IP. routinely because someone vomits when coughing.

NR. 7   SPONGIA TOSTA (SPONG.)

- See: common colds.
- The cough is ameliorated by eating or drinking something warm.

PULSATILLA NIGRICANS (PULS.)

- See: common colds.
- The cough is aggravated by lying down.
- The cough is aggravated by warmth.

BRYONIA (BRY.)

- When the chest hurts while coughing (K. p. 842: chest, pain, cough, during).
- When the chest hurts while breathing deeply and at every movement (K. p. 843: chest, pain, motion agg.).
- The pain is ameliorated by pressure and by lying on the painful side (K. p. 843: chest, pain, lying, side, painful, amel.).
- BRY. is rather warm blooded.

RANUNCULUS BULBOSUS (RAN-B.)

- Here, also the chest hurts when coughing, breathing deeply and at every movement.
- The pain is aggravated by pressure and by lying on the painful side (K. p. 843: chest, pain, lying, side, painful).
- RAN-B. are very chilly.
- RAN-B. is the most important remedy for pain under the left scapula and for herpes zoster.

SULPHUR (SULPH.)

- See: common colds.
- SULPH. is the first remedy for cough during the night.

RUMEX CRISPUS (RUMX.)

- See: common colds.
- Every change of temperature aggravates the cough.
- The cough is worst about 11 p.m.

ANTIMONIUM TARTARICUM (ANT-T.)

- See: common colds.
- ANT-T. is indicated with seriously ill patients, showing a strong cough with a lot of rattling by which the patient can't get up expectoration (d.d. STANN. who is too weak to do anything, even to talk).

D.D. cough between 2 and 4 a.m.:

- 1st remedy is KALI-C. (chilly).
- With a warm-blooded person: SULPH.
- KALI-S. are warm blooded and resemble PULS. very much.
- KALI-N.: especially with asthma in warm-blooded children.

REMEDIES AND THEIR CHARACTERISTIC SYMPTOMS IN GASTRITIS

PAPER CASE: BELLADONNA

Consultation

- A 50-year-old man, who has been treated homœopathically for his
  ulcers for 5 years, suddenly has serious stomach troubles, as if
  someone is stabbing with a knife in his stomach. The pain goes
  from the stomach to between the shoulder blades. The patient
  can't move for the pain. He perspires, suffers from heart
  palpitations, has a dry mouth, is anxious, has a warm head and
  face, with very cold feet, and wants to drink lemonade.

Discussion by Vassilis

- This is a clear picture of BELL., but also of a <u>PERFORATION OF
  THE STOMACH</u>. Here, you must be very careful. The patient
  must be hospitalized. An X-ray will show air in the abdomen. If
  you give BELL., it is possible that the pain will disappear
  temporarily but afterwards the patient will collapse with
  peritonitis.
- You can get the same picture with <u>ACUTE PANCREATITIS</u>,
  which mostly goes together with vomiting and fever.
- Vassilis mentioned this example to show that, as a homœopath,
  you must never forget the classical medical knowledge.

NR. 1   KALI CARBONICUM (KALI-C.)

- Is the most common remedy for stomach troubles.
- They display stinging and stabbing pains in the epigastrium which is very sensitive.
- Mostly, they are flatulent.
- The patient sometimes has the feeling as if his stomach is full of water (K. p. 540: stomach, water, sensation as if full of).
- There is an aggravation at night between 2 and 4 a.m., the so-called hunger-time (K. p. 1343: night, midnight after 2 to 4 a.m.).
- They can show an intense fear which comes from the stomach. (K. p. 47: fear, stomach, arising from; K. p. 476: stomach, anxiety). If the fear dominates, rather give ARS.
- The stomach troubles can start when they are overheated and then drink cold drinks (K. p. 512: stomach pain, cold drinks after, when overheated). Also after boiled fish and meat.
- They are irritable and the centre of their irritability is in the stomach: there, they feel everything, even talking (K. p. 526: stomach sensitiveness to talking).
- They are very chilly and very sensitive to the least draft of air. (K. p. 1344: air, draft agg.)
- This is the most important remedy for swellings round the eyes (K. p. 267: eye, swollen lids, œdematous). If you see this, always inquire about the night hours, even if the patient only gets up between 2 and 4 a.m. to urinate.

NR. 2   PHOSPHORUS (PHOS.)

- In case of acute stomach troubles, PHOS. desires ice-cold drinks (K. p. 512: stomach, pain, cold drinks amel.). When the drinks become warm in the stomach, the patient gets nausea or has to vomit (K. p. 532: stomach vomiting, drinking after, soon as water becomes warm in stomach). (VERAT. and BISM. display this symptom too).
- The stomachache is ameliorated by eating ice cream or cold food and drink (K. p. 513: stomach, pain, ice cream, after, amel.).

Ice-cold drinks give vasoconstriction and protect PHOS. for their serious tendency to bleedings.
- PHOS. likes fish (there is PHOS. in it) and salt. They can get gastritis by too much salt.
- In case of stomach troubles, PHOS. will become very anxious.
- PHOS. easily has stomach bleedings; then, they vomit something which looks like coffee grounds (K. p. 537: stomach, vomiting, coffee grounds, like).

NR. 3   ARSENICUM ALBUM (ARS.)

- The worst time is at night between 1 and 3 a.m. (K. p. 1343: night, midnight, after, 1 a.m.).
- The pain is mostly burning, but you can't base your prescription on that.
- The stomachache of ARS. is ameliorated after milk. If a patient says, "Milk is the best remedy for my stomach", in 99 % of the cases this is ARS. The milk can be warm or cold and must not necessarily be sweet (K. p. 514: stomach, pain, milk, after, sweet milk amel.).
- ARS. is aggravated by cold drinks, by ice cream (K. p. 513: stomach, pain, ice cream, after), by spoiled cheese or pepper sausages (K. p. 1364: food, sausages, spoiled agg.). ARS.'s complaints can start after spoiled ice cream in the summer.
- ARS. is ameliorated by warm drinks.
- They can develop an acute gastritis after having eaten sour or vinegar (K. p. 1364: food, sour agg.).
- They are very thirsty, but are continuously drinking with little sips (K. p. 529: stomach, thirst, small quantities for, often).
- Sometimes, they are sick from seeing or smelling any food.
- They can get nausea or vomiting from eating or drinking. After vomiting, they may faint (K. p. 1361: faintness, vomiting, after).
- ARS. is always chilly, they feel as cold as ice.
- They are easily exhausted, they sometimes can't vomit any more because of their weakness.
  With the combination "gastritis + vomiting + very exhausted", always think of ARS first.

- In every acute disease of ARS, you will see the well-known restlessness and fears.
- Stomach troubles which are aggravated by yawning is a keynote of ARS. (K. p. 515: stomach, pain, yawning agg). Stomach pain which is relieved by yawning often indicates LYC.

NR. 4   NUX VOMICA (NUX-V.)

- If the stomach pain is ameliorated by warm applications, this is rather a sign for NUX-V. (K. p. 515: stomach, pain, warm applications amel.) than for ARS. (K. p. 513: stomach, pain, heat amel.; stomach, pain, heat, during) (d.d. MAG-P.).
- Also the amelioration of the stomachache by warm drinks is more a sign for NUX-V than for ARS. (K. p. 515: stomach, pain, warm drinks amel.).
- NUX-V. is mostly irritable because of the pain. They like alcoholic drinks, coffee, stimulants, etc. Afterwards, they can get stomach troubles by intoxication or excess.
- NUX-V. easily develops a sensation as if there is a stone or an egg in the stomach (K. p. 527: stomach, stone, sensation of, eating, after).
- NUX-V. can get stomach bleeding by suppression of hemorrhoids (K. p. 537: stomach, vomiting blood, suppressed hemorrhoidal flow, after).
- If alcoholic people complain about hiccough, think of NUX-V. (d.d. RAN-B.: K. p. 502: stomach, hiccough, alcoholic drinks, after).

CALCAREA CARBONICA (CALC.)

- Lying on the back is the only thing that relieves the pain in case of acute gastritis (K. p. 513: stomach, pain, lying on back amel.).
- The patient feels a kind of trembling in the stomach (K. p. 530: stomach, trembling).

ELAPS CORALLINUS (ELAPS.)

- Lying on the stomach is the only thing to ease the pain in case of an acute gastritis (K. p. 513: stomach, pain, lying on abdomen amel.).
- Cold water in the stomach is experienced as ice cold (K.p. 482: stomach coldness, cold drinks, after; K. p. 483: stomach, coldness, ice, like, after cold drinks).

CHELIDONIUM MAJUS (CHEL.)

- Stool ameliorates the stomach troubles: they constantly want to go to the toilet (K. p. 514: stomach, pain, stool, after, amel.) (d.d. NAT-S.).
- The stomach pain is better when they lie down on their side (especially the left side) with the legs drawn up against the stomach (K. p. 514: stomach, pain, lying, side, left, with legs drawn up, amel.).
- The gastric pain can extend to the right shoulder blade, mostly transversely (K. p. 515: stomach, pain, extending transversely).
- The stomachache is better after warm milk (K. p. 515: stomach, pain, warm milk amel.) (d.d. ARS).
- Aggravation time of CHEL. is 4 a.m. (K. p. 1343: night, midnight, after, 4 a.m.).
- CHEL. generally likes hot drinks.
- CHEL. is generally better after eating.
- They mostly have offensive breath and a yellow tongue (K. p. 402: mouth, discoloration tongue yellow).

LYCOPODIUM CLAVATUM (LYC.)

- Most characteristic of LYC. is the sensation of fullness, the swollen stomach, and the intestinal rumbling (K. p. 498: stomach fullness, eating, even so little, after).
- They have eructations which start in the stomach, go to the pharynx and stop there. (Thus, LYC. are not always better with eructations).
- They can have a burning feeling in the pharynx that stays there for hours.
- Sometimes, they have persistent sour eructations.
- Sometimes, they have no appetite during the day, but a ravenous appetite at night (K. p. 477: stomach, appetite, increased, night).
- The hours of aggravation are 4 to 8 p.m. (K. p. 1342: afternoon 4 to 8 p.m.) and 2 a.m. (K. p. 512: stomach, pain, night, 2 a.m.) (d.d. SULPH. aggravation from 4 to 6 p.m. or from 4 to 8 p.m.).
- The stomach trouble of LYC. is worse after eating rotten fruit (K. p. 513: stomach, pain, fruit, after) or after onions (K. p. 1363: food, onion agg.), beans (K. p. 1362: food, beans and peas agg.),oysters (K. p. 1363: food, oysters agg.) and flatulent food (K. p. 1363: food, flatulent food agg.).
- The stomach pain is ameliorated by rubbing on the stomach (K. p. 514: stomach, pain, rubbing amel.).
- LYC. is thirsty for warm drinks, and only drinks small quantities at a time (K. p.529: stomach, thirst, small quantities, for).

SULPHUR (SULPH.)

- Most characteristic of SULPH. is the sour sensation. They have sour eructations, and heartburn which is aggravated by milk (K. p. 514: stomach, pain, milk, after).
- The stomachache gets worse while standing (K. p. 514: stomach, pain, standing, while) just as, with SULPH., everything gets worse while standing.

DIOSCOREA VILLOSA (DIOS.)

- Is especially seen in children who have stomach or abdominal colics: the pain is relieved only when they sit erect (K. p. 514: stomach, pain, sitting erect amel.) or stand erect or walk around (K. p. 515: stomach, pain, walking amel.). Sometimes, d.d. with CHAM. is difficult because the child is also better when you carry it, because at that moment it is upright on the arm.
- The stomach pain is relieved by bending backwards (K. p. 556: abdomen, pain, bending backwards amel.).
- Is also used for stomachache in pregnant women (K. p. 514: stomach, pain, pregnancy, during), especially if the pain gets worse while sitting bent over and stops when sitting erect or walking around with the back bent backwards with the abdomen forward.

GRAPHITES (GRAPH.)

- The most characteristic symptom is that the pain stops temporarily after eating (K. p. 513: stomach, pain, eating after, amel.)
- The stomachache is ameliorated by warm drinks and warm milk (K. p. 515: stomach, pain, warm drinks amel.; warm milk amel.)(d.d. CHEL.).
- The gastric pain can begin after eating lots of sweets, salt or fish (the aversions of GRAPH.: K. p. 480: stomach, aversion fish; K. p. 482: aversion salt food; aversion sweets).
- The stomach troubles are better by eructations (K. p. 513: stomach, pain, eructations amel.) and by lying (K. p. 513: stomach, pain, lying amel.).
- Generally, GRAPH. likes warm drinks.

COLOCYNTHIS (COLOC.)

- They produce acute stomach troubles after emotional excitement (faster than IGN.) , after anger and irritability, after torment and vexation, after mortification (K. 513: stomach, pain, anger, after; K 513: stomach, pain, excitement, after).
- They have to push very hard on their stomach (K. p. 514: stomach, pain, pressure amel.) or have to lie or sit bent double to ease the pain (K. p. 512: stomach, pain, bending double amel.).
- They have more appetite when they have a stomachache.
- They can get stomach troubles after eating potatoes (K. p. 514: stomach pain potatoes after).
- They often have a bitter taste in the mouth (K. p. 422: mouth, taste, bitter).
- Very often, the remedy STAPH. is hidden behind COLOC. COLOC. follows well after CAUST.

   d.d. IGN.: The empty feeling in the stomach does not go away by eating, they keep on eating because they never feel satisfied (K 488: stomach, emptiness, eating, not relieved by).

BRYONIA ALBA (BRY.)

- The most characteristic symptom is that every movement aggravates the pain (K. p. 514: stomach, pain, motion on).
- The patient lies quiet in bed without moving.
- Vomiting is very bad for him, and is almost unbearable.
- They can get sick or vomit even by moving their eyes.
- They have a dry mouth and are very thirsty (K. p. 403: mouth, dryness, thirst, with).
- They are irritable, don't want anyone near them (K. p. 37: disturbed, averse to being).
- After eating, they have a sensation as if there is a stone in the stomach (K. p. 527: stomach, stone, sensation, eating, after).
- The stomach troubles of BRY. are aggravated by: beans (K. p. 1362: food, beans and peas agg.), cabbages (K. p. 1362: food, cabbage agg.), bread with butter (K. p. 512: stomach, pain, bread, after), wine (K. p. 515: stomach, pain, wine, after).

PULSATILLA (PULS.)

- The stomach troubles start or are aggravated by fat or rich food (K. p. 513: stomach pain, fat food after; K. p. 514: stomach, pain rich food, after). Sometimes, the troubles start on holidays by eating too fat food or by eating pork.
- Greasy food makes them get a bad taste in their mouth and they get ill from it.
- They sometimes have a dry mouth and even so, they are THIRST-LESS, (K. p. 404: mouth, dryness, thirstless), they drink very little (K. p. 530: stomach, thirstless).
- They are mostly warm blooded, although they sometimes feel a cold sensation on the back (K. p. 885: back, coldness, extending down back).

IPECACUANHA (IP.)

- Is well-indicated for nausea during pregnancy, on condition that the nausea is the main symptom. (if pain in the stomach is the main symptom during pregnancy, think of DIOS.).
- In case of stomach troubles, with nausea and even with vomiting, the tongue stays clean and is not furred.
(See Boericke p. 352 "stomach")

ARGENTUM NITRICUM (ARG-N.)

- Characteristic is the aggravation by sweets (K. p. 1364: food, sweets agg.; d.d. IGN.).
- They sometimes have difficulty in starting to burp, and if they succeed, it is so loud that they are ashamed of it (K. p. 495: eructations, loud).

- They can have very loud intestinal rumblings or very loud flatulence (K. p. 618: rectum, flatus, loud, sugar, after).
- ARG-N. is a warm-blooded remedy.

CARBO VEGETABILIS (CARB-V.)

- They can collapse or become short of breath because of the flatulence which pushes up the diaphragm (K. p. 769: respiration, difficult, flatulence, from).
- All their complaints are ameliorated by eructations (K. p. 513: stomach, pain, eructations amel.).
- With the tendency to faint, they may begin to perspire, get blue lips and face, and with this they have a strong need for fresh air.

NATRUM CARBONICUM (NAT-C.)

- Can't support the slightest touch of the stomach.
  (K. p. 515: stomach, pain, touch)

SANGUINARIA (SANG.)

- The stomach pain is generally accompanied by vomiting and pain above the right eye (K. p. 159: head pain forehead eyes above right).
- The headache is better after vomiting (K. p. 150: head pain vomiting amel.) but the stomachache is worse by vomiting.

LOBELIA (LOB.)

- Here, vomiting will come up in attacks.
- There is a strong nausea.
- The patient is very anxious (d.d. ARS.).

PHOSPHORICUM ACIDUM

- The stomach pain comes up after excessive sexual activity (K. p. 512: stomach pain coition after).
- PH-AC. can have vertigo, headache or heart palpitations by too much sex.

REMEDIES AND THEIR CHARACTERISTIC SYMPTOMS IN CYSTITIS

NR. 1   SARSAPARILLA (SARS.)

- With SARS., you will be successful in 50 to 60 % of the cases with acute cystitis (of course, always on the condition that there is no other polychrest indicated and that it is the only complaint.).
- The necessary characteristic symptoms for SARS. are:
  1. frequent, abundant urination
  2. severe, burning pain at the end of urination
     (K. p. 673: urethra, pain, urination, at close of)
- There may be blood in the urine (K. p. 681: urine, bloody, last part, mixed with blood and pus).
- Sometimes, the bladder is very sensitive and there is a continuous urge to urinate.
- Sometimes, the patient has the feeling that air is passing through the urethra during urination (K. p. 669: urethra, air passes from the female urethra, during urination).
- The patient can be chilly as well as warm blooded. If he is extremely chilly, you'd rather give NUX-V.
- If a kidney stone comes down to the bladder and the pain is only located in the bladder, there is a great possibility that SARS. will help to pass the stone (K. p. 645: bladder, calculi). SARS. can be very useful after kidney stones which were taken away or after lithotomy (d.d. STAPH.).

- Sometimes, the cystitis is the result of being exposed to coldness or humidity (K. p. 658: bladder, urination, frequent, exposure to cold and wet).
- Urine can be slimy or sandy (K. p. 689: urine, sediment, mucous; K. p. 690: urine, sediment, sand).
- SARS. can also be used for children, weeping before or during urination (K. p. 94: weeping, micturition, before; K. p. 654: bladder, urging, painful, child cries).
- For chronic cystitis, SARS. is not indicated as the first remedy.

NR. 2 NUX VOMICA (NUX-V.)

- The most characteristic symptom is that warmth and warm applications relieve the pain and the urinary frequency (a warm bath, the warmth of the bed as well as hot drinks). ARS. has this symptom too, but it is less indicated for cystitis; it is more indicated for paralysis of the bladder.
- NUX-V. has the feeling that the bladder is always full. They often go to the toilet, and always urinate a little bit. They have the feeling that they must urinate a lot, but only a few drops will pass, while they keep on feeling that the bladder is full (K. p. 654: bladder, urging, ineffectual). If there is in addition urge to stool (whether or not ineffectual), it certainly is NUX-V.
- If they make stool, there is always a strong urge to urinate. (K. p. 634: rectum, urging, urination, during)
- NUX-V. has to urinate very often and there is pain before, during as well as after urination. Yet, the worst bladder pain is during urination. Even while making stool, the bladder pain is worse.
- The bladder feels irritated, sometimes there is a spasm of the sphincter of the bladder which is ameliorated by warm applications.
- NUX-V. is very chilly.

NR. 3   NATRIUM-CARBONICUM (NAT-C.)

- NAT-C. is especially indicated for chronic cystitis.
- They develop a burning pain in the urethra and at the end of urination and afterwards (K. p. 675: urethra, pain, burning, urination, after, close at).
- You can also think of NAT-C. if there is no result with SARS. or NUX-V. in case of an acute cystitis, especially frequently relapsing cystitis.

CANTHARIS (CANTH.)

- Most characteristic is the strong intensity of the complaints: strong burning and stabbing pain, strong urge to urinate.
- Mostly, there are sexual problems: painful erection (K. p. 695: genitalia, erection, painful) or voluptuous feelings in the vagina with desire to make love (K. p. 716: desire increased).
- Even children may show priapism with blood in the urine (K. p. 681: urine, bloody). They have such a pain that they dance around and shriek.
- Sometimes, pure drops of blood are leaving the urethra without urine.
- While drinking, the patient can feel that the drinks are doing harm to the bladder (K. p. 646: bladder, pain, drinking agg.).
- Contrary to ARS. and especially to NUX-V., the burning bladder pain of CANTH. will be ameliorated by cold applications.

PETROSELINUM (PETROS.)

- The most characteristic symptom is the <u>itching, deep in the urethra, together with itching and tingling on the perineum</u>. The itching can be voluptuous.
  (K. p. 672: urethra, itching, fossa navicularis; K. p. 680: urethra, tingling).
- Very often, there is a sudden urge to urinate (K. p. 655: bladder, urging, sudden).
- Sometimes, there is a milky discharge from the urethra (d.d. MED.). PETROS. can be used for gonorrhœa if MED. doesn't help or as a complementary remedy after MED. (K. p. 670: urethra discharge, gonorrhœal).

SEPIA (SEP.)

- They stay close to the toilet, because they have <u>continuously the feeling that they will lose urine</u>.
- They often have the sensation as if the uterus is coming out or a bearing down sensation (K. p. 736: genitalia, female, pain, bearing down uterus, urging to urinate, on). In an acute situation, you will find that they want to cross their legs or hold their abdomen in order to keep away those unpleasant feelings.
- In case of uterine prolapse with recurrent cystitis, you must think of SEP.
- SEP. will always <u>weep</u> when they are very ill. They are always very <u>chilly</u> then (if a warm blooded person weeps a lot, think of PULS.).
- SEP. often suffers from cystitis every month, just before or during the menses.
- The urine can smell like mice (K. p. 687: urine, odor, sourish).

EQUISETUM HYEMALE (EQUIS.)

- Most characteristic is a very obtuse pain and a <u>sensation of fullness in the bladder which is not ameliorated</u> by urinating. (K. p. 645: bladder, fullness).
- This remedy works well during <u>pregnancy</u> if they have this sensation of fullness and walk constantly to the toilet without losing this sensation.
- EQUIS. can be used for children with bed-wetting, on condition that nothing else but <u>pure habit</u> can be found, they are too lazy (K. p. 659: bladder, urination, involutary, night, tangible, cause except, habit, when there is no).

PHOSPHORICUM ACIDUM (PH-AC.)

- If the cystitis <u>goes together with a tremendous weakness</u>, we think of ACIDUM-remedies like PH-AC.
- The urine looks like milk, the patient urinates abundantly. (K. p. 686: urine, milky)
- The patient only wants fruit or fruit juice (be careful for dehydration) (K. p. 485: stomach, desires juicy things).

UVA URSI (UVA.)

- In case of <u>uterine prolapse with chronic bladder irritation.</u>
- There is copious urination and a pressing pain at the neck of the bladder after urination. (This remedy should be added to the repertory for its bladder symptoms)

TEREBINTHINA OLEUM (TER.)

- This is an oil which is used to make paint.
- Vassilis had a patient who was an artist and had the habit of licking his brush. He was suffering from blood in his urine (K. p. 682: urine, bloody). TER. cured him completely. (SARS. and CANTH. have more frequent blood in the urine, of course).

STAPHYSAGRIA (STAPH.)

- Especially for chronic cystitis in women having bladder troubles since they were married, or with young girls since their first sexual experience (K. p. 656: bladder, urination, dysuria, married women, newly).

CLEMATIS ERECTA (CLEM.)

- In case of chronic relapsing cystitis as a result of urethral stricture (K. p. 679: urethra, stricture).

PAPER CASE : RENAL COLIC

In case of renal colic, other remedies will be necessary than in cystitis. In case of renal stones, usually several different remedies will be necessary in succeeding order, depending on the changing picture until the stone is expelled from the body.

Vassilis gives an example from his practice:

A patient with renal colic is anxious, restless, chilly and does not find a good position to lie down: he is given RHUS-T. 200. After that, he becomes more warm blooded, lies very quietly so he won't feel the pain and he has a dry mouth: he is given BRY. 200. Then, the pain is extending from his back to the groin: he is given BERB. 200. Later, there is blood in the urine and the patient has a burning pain after urination: he is given SARS. 200. The next day, the patient urinated a little stone and he was cured.

Conclusion:

In dangerous, very painful acute diseases, you have to follow the symptoms day after day and give the remedy the body is asking for at that moment.

REMEDIES AND THEIR CHARACTERISTIC SYMPTOMS IN COLITIS AND DIARRHŒA

NR. 1 PODOPHYLLUM (PODO.)

- The 2 most characteristic symptoms of PODO. are:

  1st: diarrhœa with a lot of flatus, flatulence, noise and force. If they have stool, it is like a kind of explosion of diarrhœa, so that the toilet and even the patient are dirty.

  2nd: There is a <u>sensation of emptiness in the abdomen after diarrhœa</u> (K. p. 546: abdomen, emptiness). Sometimes, they are generally exhausted and weak after diarrhœa, so that they have the feeling they will faint or die (K. p. 1416: weakness, diarrhœa, from; d.d. ARS.).

- The diarrhœa of PODO. is worst in the morning. They have to go to the toilet sometimes 10 times one after the other and then not again during the rest of the day (K. p. 610: rectum, diarrhœa, forenoon).
- Very often, there are intestinal rumblings and flatulence.
- Frequently, there is abdominal pain, which is aggravated by bending, bending double, pressure and warm applications, but is ameliorated by lying on the stomach.

- PODO. is a strong remedy for rectal prolapse. Think of it in case of diarrhœa, during vomiting and in children (K. p. 631: rectum, prolapsus, diarrhœa, during; prolapsus, vomiting, when; prolapsus, children).
- The centre of the pathology with PODO. is situated in the gall-bladder and the liver (K. p. 568: pain, liver). If, in case of stinking diarrhœa with explosive spluttering stool, you have to chose between SULPH. and PODO., rather take PODO. for adults and SULPH. for children (children do not have as many liver troubles as adults do).
- For diarrhœa in AIDS patients, you may also think of PODO.
- PODO. is not very well worked out in the repertory. Diarrhœa used to appear more in case of cholera and therefore, CAMPH. was more indicated at that time.
- PODO. is the strongest remedy for diarrhœa after having eaten oysters (K. p. 614: rectum, diarrhœa, oysters, after).

NR. 2 VERATRUM ALBUM (VERAT.)

- The characteristic symptoms of VERAT. are:

1. Combination of vomiting and diarrhœa (K. p. 532: vomiting, diarrhœa, during). diarrhœa is copious, frequent, with violence and goes together with colic pains and abdominal cramps.

2. Cold perspiration on forehead during or after diarrhœa (K. p. 1297: perspiration, diarrhœa, with).

3. Cold sensation on abdomen or stomach (K. p. 542: abdomen, coldness). Even the tongue and breath can be cold. (K. p. 399: mouth, cold breath; cold tongue).

- With a combination of these characteristic symptoms, you should give VERAT. and not ARS., even if the patient is anxious. Sometimes, d.d. with ARS. is difficult.
- VERAT. is thirsty for cold drinks.

NR. 3 CUPRUM (CUPR.)

- The characteristic symptoms of CUPR. are:

1. Intestinal cramps with nausea, diarrhœa and cold extremities.

2. A warm sensation on the abdomen (K. p. 551: abdomen, heat).

- CUPR. is the greatest remedy for cramps in the whole body. With diarrhœa, there will always be intestinal cramps or colic pains. If there is diarrhœa together with cramps wherever in the body, do think of CUPR. With CUPR., intestinal cramps will occur especially after the diarrhœa.
- With CUPR., everything is ameliorated by drinking cold water (see Boericke p. 248 "CUPR. modalities"). That's why even the cramps and the nausea will be ameliorated by drinking something cold.
- The intestinal cramps get worse by moving. If the patient moves, the cramps come back very violently. In case of diarrhœa with such a modality, firstly think of CUPR. and secondly of BRY.
- CUPR. is mostly warm blooded.

NR. 4 ARSENICUM ALBUM (ARS.)

- Characteristic is the strong weakness and exhaustion, even in case of a slight diarrhœa, i.e. the strong exhaustion is not in proportion to the small quantity of stool. ARS. may even faint after diarrhœa (K. p. 1359: faintness diarrhœa after) or after vomiting (K. p. 1361: faintness vomiting after).
VERAT. and PODO. must have had large quantities of diarrhœa before they will be exhausted.
- ARS. has to make stool continuously but always a little bit. The diarrhœa is dark and offensive.
- Cold drinks or cold food aggravate the diarrhœa, that's why they usually prefer other things (K. p. 611: rectum, diarrhœa, cold drinks, after; K. p. 613: diarrhœa, food, cold, agg.) (d.d. DULC.).

- ARS. can develop a colitis from anxiety (K. p. 611: rectum, diarrhœa, anxiety, after), while the rectum burns like fire and the pain is relieved by warm applications. This applies diarrhœa as well as piles. The anus is easily excoriated in case of diarrhœa. The colitis of ARS. will always go together with anxiety about health.
- ARS. is very chilly and very thirsty, but drinks frequently with little sips (K. p. 529: stomach, thirst, small quantities, often).
- An ARS. colitis is mostly very bad, and can easily produce sepsis (K. p. 615: rectum diarrhœa septic conditions, from). Hospitalization can be necessary in such cases.

SULPHUR (SULPH.)

- Characteristic is the offensive diarrhœa, like spoiled eggs (K. p. 618: rectum, flatus, offensive, spoiled eggs; K. p. 640: stool, odor, eggs, like rotten). SULPH. is more frequent than ARN. with this symptom. It is a keynote of SULPH.
- Characteristic is also the itching of the rectum (K. p. 622: rectum, itching, burning). Both in chronic and acute cases. Sometimes, it is a burning sensation, which is ameliorated by cold applications (d.d. ALOE.). The itching of the rectum is aggravated by contact with water or by taking a bath.
- Often they must get up at night because of the diarrhœa, mostly at 5 a.m. (K. p. 610: rectum, diarrhœa, morning, waking with urging 5 a.m.).
- The colitis can start or get worse after beer (d.d. ALOE.) (K. p. 611: rectum, diarrhœa, beer, after).
- For children, SULPH. is the first remedy in case of an acute diarrhœa, for adults, the first remedy is PODO. (see PODO.).
- In case of diarrhœa, there is very often the characteristic pain in the forehead, ameliorated by cold applications (K. p. 156: head, pain, forehead, cold applications amel.). SULPH. is mostly warm blooded. They have an offensive perspiration and are thirsty.
- SULPH.'s diarrhœa can start by suppression of eruptions e.g. with cortisone ointment (K. p. 612: rectum, diarrhœa, eruptions suppressed, after) (d.d. PSOR. and DULC.).

ALOE (ALOE.)

- Characteristic is that the patient, when he has diarrhœa, continuously has to think of his rectal sphincter. They constantly have the feeling as if they will lose stool, especially if they break wind (K. p. 621: rectum, involuntary stool, flatus, on passing). They are not able to feel the difference between wind and soft stool. It makes them very irritable. They don't want anybody with them, they feel bored. If they talk to somebody and their attention goes away from the sphincter for a moment, they will lose stool involuntary.
- Involuntary loss of stool with flatus in children makes you think of ALOE., in older people of HYOS. or GAMB.
- The flatulence sometimes feels very hot (K. p. 618: rectum, flatus, hot).
- The diarrhœa of ALOE. can start after beer (K. p. 611: rectum, diarrhœa, beer, after), oysters or crustaceans (K. p. 614: rectum, diarrhœa, oysters, after).
- Sometimes, they must get up at 5 a.m. because of the diarrhœa. (K. p. 1255: sleep, waking, 5 a.m., with urging to stool).
- Sometimes, ALOE.'s stool looks like small hard balls swimming in a watery fluid.

- D.d. ALOE.-SULPH.:

    Is sometimes very difficult. They have a lot of similar symptoms: offensive diarrhœa, diarrhœa after beer, burning pain in rectum during stool and cold applications ameliorate, diarrhœa at 5 a.m. (K. p. 609 and 1255).
    The differences are: ALOE.'s rectum is dry, SULPH.'s is wet. The anal complaints of ALOE. are ameliorated by cold applications, while SULPH. can't bear water and thus can be aggravated by it. With ALOE., you'll find the uncertain feeling in the anus while with SULPH., there is an offensive odor and/or an odor of spoiled eggs.

RHUS TOXICODENDRON (RHUS-T.)

- Diarrhœa after getting wet (K. p. 615: rectum, diarrhœa, wet, after getting), e.g. a child playing in the rain gets diarrhœa afterwards (here, do think of DULC. too).
- They sometimes have to get up at 4 a.m. with diarrhœa (K. p. 610: rectum, diarrhœa, night, midnight, after, 4 a.m.), sometimes accompanied by anxiety, chilliness or fever.

CAMPHORA (CAMPH.)

- Most characteristic is the serious diarrhœa in an ice-cold patient, who nevertheless doesn't want to be covered (K. p. 1275: chill, uncovering amel.). The patient is very chilly and the skin feels very cold. Even the tongue and breath are cold (K. p. 399: mouth, cold breath; cold tongue).
- Peculiar of CAMPH. is that the patient doesn't want to be covered in spite of the coldness, and wants to be covered in spite of the warmth (K. p. 1275: chill, uncovered wants to be with cold dry skin, but desire to be covered with heat and sweat).

MERCURIUS CORROSIVUS (MERC-C.)

- Most characteristic is the sensation that stool is hot (K. p. 638: stool, hot) and that there is mostly blood during stool (K. p. 636: stool, bloody).
- There is also a strong urge to stool (K. p. 630: rectum, pain, tenesmus, diarrhœa, during) in case of diarrhœa. They constantly go to the toilet to make a bit of stool and immediately afterwards the urge comes back (d.d. NUX-V).

- If the patient perspires offensively, has offensive breath and salivates during the sleep, give MERC-SOL.
- In case of a serious ulcerative colitis, think of MERC-C. as a first remedy.

GAMBOGIA (GAMB.)

- Watery diarrhœa in aged people (K. p. 610: rectum, diarrhœa, aged people).
- This is a rather rare remedy which you can use when PODO. and SULPH. have no result.
- The best indication for GAMB. is continuous diarrhœa in aged people.

CROTON TIGLIUM (CROT-T.)

- Most characteristic is that the diarrhœa comes suddenly and violently, like a shot from a gun (K. p. 637: stool, forcible).
- While the patient is eating or drinking, he already gets the feeling that he must go to the toilet (K. p. 612: rectum, diarrhœa drinking, immediately after; eating after). It is as if he has the feeling that he must let out what he has just eaten.
- The diarrhœa is copious, watery and yellow-coloured.
- There is a constant urge to stool (K. p. 633: rectum, urging, constant).
- After the diarrhœa, they have nausea without being able to vomit and they sometimes get saliva in the mouth.
- There may be sudden intestinal spasms.
- The patient sometimes has the feeling that his intestines are full of water (K. p. 605: abdomen, water, as if full of). Sometimes, it sounds like a swirling river.
  (d.d. KALI-C. has the feeling that the stomach is full of water)

- CROT-T. is mostly used for cases of chronic diarrhœa. In acute situations, think of it when there is a combination of gushing acute diarrhœa and acute skin-eruptions.
- The sensitivity of temperature is not important.
- If a patient with colitis has an itching skin-eruption from the moment he eats or drinks something, you can think of CROT-T.

CARBO-VEGETABILIS (CARB-V.)

- Diarrhœa after fat and rich food in a chilly patient (K. p. 613: rectum, diarrhœa, food, fat, after).
  If the patient is warm blooded, think of PULS.
- With CARB-V., everything is better after eructations, also the diarrhœa (K. p. 612: diarrhœa, eructations, amel.).

MAGNESIA PHOSPHORICA (MAG-P.)

- They can have colitis without real diarrhœa.
- Most characteristic is the abdominal pain which is ameliorated by rubbing, because of the warmth of the hand(d.d. COLOC. no amelioration by rubbing) and is ameliorated by warm applications and warm drinks (K. p. 561: abdomen, pain, warm drinks amel.; warmth amel.).
- The patient must walk around in order to make flatus; then, he feels better.
- In the mouth, the tongue is clean as with IP.: a clean tongue in spite of the intestinal problem.

CHAMOMILLA (CHAM.)

- Characteristic is the green stool, which looks like spinach (K. p. 637: stool, green).
- They are very irritable (K. p. 58: irritability, children, in), have a red cheek (K. p. 362: face, discoloration, red, one sided, one pale the other red) and are generally better if they are carried (K. p. 10: carried, desires to be). The diarrhœa too stops when they are carried.
- CHAM. is often used with children having dentition problems. (K. p. 431: teeth, dentition, difficult).

COLOCYNTHIS (COLOC.)

- The characteristic symptom that must be present with COLOC., is the colic pain which is ameliorated by pressure and by sitting bent double (K. p. 556: abdomen, pain, bend double, must).
- diarrhœa can start after anger (K. p. 611: rectum, diarrhœa, anger, after), grief or vexation (K. p. 613: diarrhœa, grief, after; K. p. 615: diarrhœa, vexation, from). It may also start after eating potatoes (K. p. 614: diarrhœa, potatoes, after).
- COLOC. sometimes press on the abdomen with something hard to relieve the pain (K. p. 559: abdomen, pain, pressure amel.).
- The abdominal cramps are better immediatly after stool (K. p. 561: abdomen, pain, stool, after, amel.).

RHEUM (RHEUM.)

- Is an acid remedy.
  Everything smells very sour: mouth, breath, saliva, perspiration and discharge such as diarrhœa and stool (K. p. 640: stool, odor, sour).
- Can be used constitutionally or in an acute situation.

PHOSPHORICUM ACIDUM (PH-AC.)

- They can get <u>diarrhœa after taking a cold in the summer</u> (K. p. 612: rectum, diarrhœa, cold, taking cold, after, summer, in).
- Although PH-AC. is a weak remedy, the patient isn't so weakened by diarrhœa as e.g. ARS. (K. p. 615: rectum, diarrhœa, weakness, without).

PHOSPHORUS (PHOS.)

- The <u>diarrhœa can be ameliorated by cold drinks or cold food</u> (K. p. 611: diarrhœa, cold drinks amel.; K. p. 613: diarrhœa, food, cold, amel.).
- The <u>diarrhœa can dissappear after eating ice cream</u> (K. p. 613: diarrhœa, ice cream amel.).

PULSATILLA (PULS.)

- Just as everything is changeable with PULS., the diarrhœa is changeable too (K. p. 636: stool, changeable).
- The <u>diarrhœa mostly begins after rich food, fat or fried food</u> (K. p. 613: diarrhœa, food, rich, after; diarrhœa, food, fat, after) (d.d. CARB-V.). They may even get diarrhœa after having eaten pork (K. p. 614: diarrhœa, pork, after).
- The diarrhœa is aggravated in a warm environment (K. p. 615: diarrhœa, warmth agg.).

DULCAMARA (DULC.)

- The diarrhœa can begin after contact with cold, wet ground (K. p. 612: diarrhœa, cold nights; diarrhœa, cold, taking cold, after; diarrhœa, cold weather, from).
- The diarrhœa can begin by a climatic change to wet weather (K. p. 612: diarrhœa, damp, cold weather).

BRYONIA (BRY.)

- Every movement causes diarrhœa.

NOTE:

If the diarrhœa goes together with the following main symptoms:

- **+ vomiting:** think first of VERAT.
- **+ colics:** think first of COLOC.
- **+ cramps:** think first of CUPR.
- **+ ice cold sensation:** think first of CAMPH.
- **+ great exhaustion:** think first of ARS.

SULPHUR : ESSENCE

SULPH. is the most frequent homœopathic remedy in practice as well as in the materia medica.

Nowadays, SULPH. is sometimes difficult to diagnose. Today, a lot of former external symptoms of SULPH. are suppressed aggressively. E.g. everything that is offensive is smoothed away or camouflaged, the dirty unwashed SULPH. aren't seen anymore because of the current hygiene, the perspiration is suppressed with deodorants and anti-perspiration remedies and every rash is treated with the most recent steroid ointments.

SULPH.'s old external signs of identification can be used less nowadays, and that's why we have to look for other signs of identification.

Today, there are mainly two totally opposed types of SULPH.

The 1st type:
The tall, slender philosophical patient who walks with his shoulders bent forwards and downwards (K. p. 1403: stoop-shouldered). He is an example of the SCIENTIST who, during his whole life, is looking for the truth: in his laboratory, surrounded by his books, or with his computer. This type has a rather low sexual desire.

The 2nd type:
The plethoric SULPH. Plethoric at every level. They have a red face and very red lips. They have greasy hair and an oily face. They are fat, because they eat and drink too much. They are social people who are seen everywhere. This type has a strong sexual desire.

THE FIRST TYPE OF SULPH.

The tall philosophical scientist is most difficult to recognize. For that reason, this type is discussed at length now.

SULPH. IS A REMEDY OF POLARITIES

In the same life, SULPH. can be very fastidious for a whole period (as much as NUX-V. or ARS.) and then, for a whole period very lazy. They may show such polarities in every field, psychologically as well as in their character or in their physical appearance.
This polarity can be found with one single patient as well as with several different SULPH.-patients.

E.g.:

- one is slovenly, the other fastidious (K. p. 42: fastidious: you can add SULPH. 2nd degree).
- one is inert, the other over-enthusiastic.
- one is lazy, the other a workaholic.
- one is selfish, the other unselfish.
- one has an urge for sweets (K. p. 486: desire sweets), the other an aversion to sweets (K. p. 82: aversion sweets).
- one desires fat, the other has stomach troubles because of the fat (K. p. 487: stomach, disordered from fat).

SULPH. IS A SEEKER OF "THE TRUTH"

The scientist wants to find the truth, the deeper sense of life and the world. They read all existing books, they study every theory. They can look for the truth in mathematics for many years, or for the causative agent of a certain disease. Sometimes, they are so absorbed in their study that they totally neglect their appearance: hair uncombed, ragged clothing (K. p. 55: indifference personal appearance). You can see them walk around with piles of books in their arms, and in their office or room, you will stumble over the books that are all over the place.
We may even be talking about the "eccentric scientist" who pays attention to nothing but his study (K. p. 48: foolish behaviour, happiness and pride).
However, the problem is that everything changes and alters through time. That's what our seeker of the truth mostly will find out after some years. If SULPH. is disillusioned by a certain theory or if they find out that there is no single truth, they may suddenly let go of everything and change to something completely different. Or they will throw away all former theories and start explaining things in an esoteric way. They will sometimes start meditating in order to find the truth in another way (K. p. 87: theorizing).

SULPH. HAS A STRONG NEED OF RECOGNITION

SULPH. doesn't work for the money or to become rich, but they do it for the recognition they finally want to get. They hope their name will be known and praised because of their invention or their new theory. In their innermost being, they are convinced that the outer world will give them the recognition they deserve, considering the great deal of work they had done to seek "the truth". When they are older, they hope that they can write books with all the truths they have found and that they will get recognition.
The only thing SULPH. wants for his work is RECOGNITION. Everybody must know that they are the best.

It is a good thing that their surroundings say they admire and appreciate them, because only then they feel good. When SULPH. don't get the recognition they think they deserve, they feel bad, are closed, they withdraw into themselves, want to be alone and don't want to talk to anybody, they feel misunderstood by their environment. This may lead to melancholy and suicidal tendencies, so that d.d. with AUR. becomes difficult. SULPH. can start drinking whisky to forget their problems (K. p. 484: desires whisky).
But, SULPH. will not easily commit suicide because in their innermost being they are too selfish and too proud.

SULPH. IS SELFISH AND EGOTISTICAL

The need for admiration and recognition is the <u>food for their EGO</u> (K. p. 39: egotism). You are SULPH.'s best friend when you tell them regularly they are not selfish.
If you are critical however, they will get the feeling that you won't give them the recognition they deserve, and they will get angry or don't want to see you anymore. Sometimes, SULPH. absolutely wants to be the most important person and the centre of a group, sometimes they want to be the teacher or the guru. Those who don't agree with them, are banished from the group.

SULPH. can have the feeling that he can't stand the comparison with others. They know so much, have studied and read so much, and if at last they publish everything they have discovered, everybody will see that they are the first and the best (K. p. 51: haughty).

Sometimes, SULPH. attaches no interest to the common daily life because everything is superficial and wrong. They withdraw into themselves in order to find the truth and the right way so they can make life and the world better. If they show up with the truth then, everything will be different and we will have a better world (= SELFISH).

SULPH. CAN BE OVER-CRITICAL

SULPH. knows a lot about everything because they have read and studied so much. They thus become critical of everybody, including their colleagues. Sometimes, it looks like jealousy, but it is not: it is being over-critical (K. p. 10: censorius, critical).
They may sometimes be so over-critical that they can never say a good word. Even if everything is alright, they will find something to criticize.

MANY HOMŒOPATHS ARE SULPH.-TYPES

E.g.: They don't want to go to another homœopath for treatment: they have the feeling that nobody will ever find the remedy they need, except themselves. They think they know what they need and thus take the complete materia medica, one remedy after the other.

E.g.: The self-sacrificing homœopath (K. p. 55: indifference, welfare of others, to) who works from morning to night, not for the money, but to save the patient. They'll do everything so the patient might say: "You are a good doctor, you are the only one who has helped me so well."

SULPH. IS THE PERSON WITH MOST DISGUST

SULPH. can be disgusted by everybody of around them (K. p. 37: disgust). They don't smell their own offensive smell, but smell everything of other people. They will never drink from the same glass as their daughter or son. The child will never drink from his sister's or brother's glass.
After shaking hands or having visited an ill patient, they wash their hands (d.d. SYPH.).

They can show a fear of diseases and microbes. If they come in contact with a contagious disease, they might throw their clothes away.
They can get nausea from the odour of their own body (K 509: nausea, odour of his own body).

SULPH. HAS A STRONG ANXIETY ABOUT OTHERS

SULPH.-men are good fathers, but if their child is ill, they can become very angry and irritable. They suffer because their child is ill. All their plans fall through because of their child's illness.
SULPH. has a strong "anxiety about others" (K. p. 7: anxiety, others, for). This strong anxiety exists because they have a STRONG IMAGINATION. They suppose all kinds of situations that might happen to their loved ones. E.g.: If SULPH. are far away from their family, they'll be afraid that something might happen and for that reason they will call home every day. E.g.: If they see a stranger or someone in the family on a high place, they may be scared to death while thinking of what might happen.
Sometimes, their imagination is so strong that they get afraid they will kill their children. They won't tell such a thing easily to a doctor, but sometimes they tell the doctor they feel they might do their children some harm. This feeling can be found very strongly in SULPH.
You can add a new rubric in the repertory: FEAR TO KILL HIS/HER CHILDREN: NUX-V., SULPH., THEA.

SULPH. CAN BE VERY LAZY AND LIKES TO THEORIZE

SULPH.-students can be lazy if they have to study. They would rather call on their friends with whom they have philosophical discussions. To theorize informally, they are not lazy: that is their own special world where they feel at home. SULPH. likes discussions such as: What is the sun, what is the vibration of energy and the cosmos, what is death and what will happen after it, what is the soul, what must happen to mankind if he is no longer, what to do with negative vibrations of others etc., etc.

If SULPH. has to study or to do homework, they begin with it, do one page and then, take an interesting book to read for an hour or two. Everybody thinks they study hard while they only do what they want to do (selfish).

SULPH. has a tendency to POSTPONE: they'll sooner put off till tomorrow what they could do today.

SULPH. CAN BECOME HYPOCRITICAL

Sometimes, SULPH. can discover that they are selfish. Then, they will occupy themselves with meditation (K. p. 64: meditation) and spiritual or supernatural things (K. p. 71: religious affection). This makes them again acquire more knowledge than others, which makes them even more selfish.

SULPH. will always be someone who needs appreciation and recognition. Sometimes, they do things which are not so real or truthful. When they experience that others therefore appreciate them, their ego will be flattered so much that they'll go on doing things like that. This way, SULPH. can become very hypocritical (you can add SULPH. 3rd degree in the repertory K. p. 52: hypocrisy). In their heart, they know that they don't really deserve this recognition, but still they go on.

THE SECOND TYPE OF SULPH.

The obese, plethoric people who enjoy all the good things that life offers.

They can be recognized by their plethoric appearance (K. p. 1391: plethora): a red face, very red lips (K. p. 363: face, discoloration, red lips), they are fat (K. p. 1376: obesity), they have a greasy, oily face.

Sometimes, they are rich people who only eat in the best restaurants surrounded by a select company. They talk to their table-companions and at the same time look around to see if the others are looking at them.

They can be very generous, give money to churches and poor people. Sometimes, they are very religious, go to churches. It looks as if they sacrifice themselves for others and everybody will see them as the kindest persons on earth. Yet, in their heart the selfish element still exists, with its need of appreciation and recognition as food for their ego. Nobody sees this selfishness. This type of SULPH. doesn't think of himself as selfish, they are convinced they are sacrificing themselves. If you tell them they are selfish, you'll be their worst enemy; if, on the other hand, you claim the opposite, you will be promoted to their best friend and they will really enjoy your compliments.
SULPH.'s partners will tell you that they are selfish. They say that SULPH. comes home late in the evening and then finishes half a bottle of whisky and theorizes for the whole evening. If the partner doesn't agree with them, they get very angry (You'll know that by the partner's history).

This type of SULPH. is <u>sexually very active</u>. They appreciate their partner very much on the condition that their partner gives them the recognition they want. If this is not so, they will search for a boy/girlfriend who does appreciate them.

This person is praised to the skies, he/she is "the most beautiful on earth", an "angel". And when you see this boy/girlfriend, he or she is the most ordinary, everyday person.

The relationship with the sexual partner is strong as long as there is recognition, but from the moment this disappears, the relationship will weaken and SULPH. can part without too many problems and look for a new partner.

That's why women with a SULPH.-husband can easily become IGN. or STAPH.

SULPH. IS FOUND LESS IN WOMEN

You'll find SULPH. more in men than in women. In women, you can find the same essence as described above. Other characteristics for women are:

- In the menopause, they weep as much as PULS. (can be added in the repertory).
- They can be nailbiters as bad as MED., especially when they are anxious.
- They often have gastritis with sour eructations during the menses (K. p. 514: stomach pain, menses, during).
- They easily have offensive leucorrhœa, yellow-coloured, with itching in the vagina.
- They sometimes develop all the symptoms of PULS., but have a strong desire for fat.

CHARACTERISTIC SYMPTOMS OF SULPH.
TO BASE YOUR PRESCRIPTION ON

SULPH. is sometimes difficult to find. They can be vegetarians who suppress their instincts so much that their desire for fat and salt disappears. Sometimes, they look at their whole life philosophically and theorize during the whole consultation. Some SULPH.-parents forbid their children to eat what they want. Sometimes, SULPH. feels better than the therapist and you really feel inferior in front of them.
For all these reasons, it is very important to know very well the priority of characteristic symptoms of SULPH.

SULPH. IS MOSTLY WARM BLOODED

They can be chilly too but even then, they will easily uncover their feet (K. p. 1013: extremities, heat, foot, burning, uncovers them). Even with cold feet, they will easily uncover them or walk bare-foot (K. p. 1222: extremities, uncover, inclination to, feet).
If the feet are burning and so are the palms of the hand, we first have to think of MED. and then of SULPH. (K. p.1005: fanned, wants hands and feet). Typical of SULPH. are the restless legs and feet, which get better by putting them out of bed or cooling them (K. p. 1188: restlessness lower limbs, leg, night, must put it out of bed to cool it).

SULPH. IS MOSTLY OFFENSIVE

"Offensiveness" gives in the differential diagnosis always more points to SULPH. than to any other remedy.

- Sometimes, they just stink during the examination.
- They have offensive breath in the morning.
- The discharge from anus or ear can stink too.
- The stool is mostly very offensive. The toilet can stink enormously if someone comes after them (sometimes, SULPH. is unaware of this).
- Offensive perspiring feet (K. p. 1183: extremities, perspiration, foot, offensive: SULPH. must be 3rd degree, stronger than KALI-C. and TELL., and as strong as LYC.).

SULPH. HAS A LOT OF ITCHING

This is on every part of the body. They sometimes get neurodermatitis from scratching. Very often, there is itching on the back of the head on the hair line (K. p. 129: head, itching, occiput); sometimes, there is also a moist eruption.
SULPH. mostly has <u>itching on ANUS or in RECTUM</u> (K. p. 622: rectum, itching, daytime). It is an unbearable itching which can extend all over the perineum. Very often, there is <u>moisture on anus</u> (K. p. 623: rectum, moisture, scratching) (d.d. ALOE.: anus and rectum are dry).

SULPH. HAS A STRONG FEAR OF HIGH PLACES

If you ask them if they are afraid of something, SULPH. will give a negative answer, they don't have any fears. When you then ask them if they have fear of heights, they will say: "Oh yes, but that is very normal!"

They mostly have vertigo if they are on a high place (K. p. 100: vertigo, high places). They sometimes have the feeling that their genitalia are pulled down when they are on a high place. SULPH. may also suffer from FEAR OF NARROW PLACES (K. p. 46: fear, narrow place, in: SULPH. may be added in the repertory beside IGN. and NAT-M.).
This makes d.d. with ARG-N. even more difficult (they both are warm blooded, desire sweet, are thirsty, extroverted and have fear of high and narrow places; ARG-N. imagines all kinds of things that might happen).

SULPH. EASILY HAS WEEKEND-HEADACHE

Never give SULPH. based only on this symptom. Always see if there is no other constitutional remedy behind it. The explanation SULPH. gives for his weekend migraine is:

"I have a headache on Sunday
- because I have nothing to do
- because I don't see my girlfriend
- because I sleep longer then (K. p. 1402: sleep, long agg.)
- because I relax."

When someone gets a headache while he relaxes, think of SULPH. first.

SULPH. easily shows a burning pain on the forehead or the vertex, ameliorated by cold applications and in open air (K. p. 156: head, pain, forehead, cold applications amel.) (d.d. PULS).

SULPH. IS AGGRAVATED BY WATER

SULPH. can get an eruption, a headache or other pains by taking a bath (K. p. 1345: bathing agg.). After bathing, they feel mostly cold and easily get a cold afterwards. Children sometimes don't want to wash themselves or weep when they have to take a bath.

SULPH. USUALLY PERSPIRES EASILY

The perspiration is offensive. Very often, SULPH. doesn't smell his own bad odour, but is irritated by the slightest smell of an other (K. p. 37: disgust).

SULPH. HAS A GENERAL AGGRAVATION ABOUT 11 A.M.

The most important symptom we will see at 11 a.m. (K. p. 1341: morning, 11 a.m.) is the empty feeling in stomach or a hungry feeling (K. p. 477: stomach, appetite, increased, forenoon 11 a.m.): they just have to eat something, otherwise they won't feel good.
In case of a headache about 10 or 11 a.m., we rather think of NAT-M, GELS., BOR. and THUJ. (K. p. 134: head, pain, forenoon 10 a.m.).

SULPH. HAS NIGHTMARES WHEN SLEEPING ON THE BACK

If a patient tells you this symptom spontaneously, you get the so-called signature of SULPH. (K. p. 1242: sleep, dreams, nightmare, lying on the back).

They sometimes don't say it so clearly. E.g.: "I can only sleep on my side, if not I'll have dreams."

SULPH. can fall asleep in every position, but very often it is left.

When SULPH. doesn't sleep very well, it will be as follows: they wake up every hour (K. p. 1256: sleep, waking frequent, midnight, after) and then sleep again (so-called cat-nap sleep). Because of this, they are not refreshed in the morning and if they sleep longer then, they'll get up with a headache.

SULPH. SOMETIMES HAS TO GET UP FROM BED WITH URGING TO STOOL

They have to get up from bed to make stool. Sometimes, it is diarrhœa. This is mostly about 5 a.m. but may be later too (K. p. 610: rectum, diarrhœa, morning, waking with urging, 5 a.m.).

SULPH. HAS BURNING AND ITCHING EYES

They have a sensation as if there is SAND IN THE EYES and they try to get it out (K. p. 258: eye, pain, sand, as from).
There is often discharge from the eyes, sometimes offensive. With children, the eyes are sometimes agglutinated in the morning.

WHAT DOES SULPH. LIKE VERY MUCH ?

- FAT and MEAT like NIT-AC., ARS., NUX-V., MED., TUB., MEZ. etc. That's why they have so much heart and vascular disease and high blood pressure (K. p. 485: stomach, desires fat).
- SWEETS: leads to a tendency to diabetes (K. p. 486: stomach, desires sweets).
  Women have an increased desire for sweet things before the menses.
- ALCOHOL, WHISKY and BEER (K. p. 484: desires beer, whisky, wine).
- Sometimes salt.
- CHOCOLATE and CUCUMBERS may be added.

WHAT DOES SULPH. DISLIKE ?

- SOUR: SULPH. is mentioned 2nd degree with "aversion and desire sour" (K. p. 480: aversion to acids; K. p. 486: desire sour, acids). With d.d. between SULPH. and MED., you can use this point. MED. mostly has a strong desire for sour, so with "aversion acids", rather give SULPH.
- EGGS (K. p. 480: aversion eggs).
- FISH (K. p. 480: aversion fish).
- AVERSION CHICKEN: You can add this rubric on K. p. 480 with NAT-M. 3rd degree, SULPH. 2nd degree.
- AVERSION OLIVES: You can add this rubric on K. p. 482 with SULPH. 3rd degree (in the rubric desires olives: add SULPH. 2nd degree: SULPH. is the remedy of polarities).

WHAT WILL TROUBLE SULPH. ?

- SULPH. is aggravated by MILK (K. p. 1363: food, milk agg.).
- SULPH. is aggravated by HONEY.

Mostly, it will give SULPH. stomach troubles. The most frequent stomach trouble is a burning sensation that goes into the oesophagus.

SULPH. CAN'T STAND UPRIGHT FOR A PROLONGED TIME

SULPH. likes to lie down in an easy chair. Every symptom is aggravated by standing, e.g. psychological, pain in the back (K. p. 898: back, pain, standing, while), stomach troubles (K. p. 514: stomach, pain, standing, while), etc. SULPH. doesn't like to saunter, doesn't like to buy and try on clothes.

SULPH. GETS DISEASES FROM THE SUPPRESSION OF ERUPTIONS

By continued treatment of eczema with steroid cortisone ointments, they can get a headache (K. p. 149: head, pain, suppressed eruptions) or asthma (K. p. 765: respiration, asthmatic, eruptions, after suppressed).

SULPH. IS A NAILBITER

- Nailbiting is not so strong in SULPH. as in MED.

SULPH. CAN LAUGH DURING SLEEP

In the rubric "K. p. 62: laughing, sleep, during", you can make
SULPH. 3rd degree, like LYC.

DIFFERENTIAL DIAGNOSIS OF SULPH.

ARGENTUM NITRICUM (ARG-N.)

They are both warm blooded, have a fear of heights and narrow
places, are thirsty, desire sweets and salt, are extroverted.

- If they have many troubles because of sweets, rather think of
  ARG-N. (K. p. 1364: food, sweets agg.).
- The combination very strong desire for sweets and salt (K. p. 486:
  desire salt) makes you rather think of ARG-N.
- If the combination desire sweets and fat is very strong, rather
  think of SULPH.
- The combination desire sweets and aversion fat: rather ARG-N.
- If they uncover their feet, rather think of SULPH. If they don't,
  think of ARG-N.
- If there is itching and offensive smell, rather think of SULPH.
- In case of lumbago, the pain in the back of ARG-N. is better by
  standing, of SULPH. worse by standing (K. p. 898: back, pain,
  standing, while, amel.).

MEDORRHINUM (MED.)

- In MED., all desires are MUCH STRONGER than in SULPH. If you have a person with a very strong desire for fat, salt, alcohol, spicy food, sweets, sour and sour fruit, think first of MED.
- Sometimes, the essence is not clear, they can both be sexually very active and MED. must not necessarily be cruel. Moreover, making a differential diagnosis on desires and aversions is difficult.
- With aversion sour, think more of SULPH.
- In case of a very strong fear of high places or a clear aggravation about 11 a.m., rather think of SULPH.
- If the ankles are swollen, rather think of MED. (K. p. 1201: swelling ankle).
- Characteristic of MED. is the feeling or the fear someone is behind or beside them, especially in the dark (K. p. 43: fear, behind him, that someone is; fear dark).
- A big difference between SULPH. and MED. is that with SULPH., everything is aggravated at night, e.g. cough, pain in left shoulder, eruption, itching.
  MED. on the other hand, is better at night: they are real night-people (K. p. 1342: evening amel.).
- With a combination of urethritis or cystitis with conjunctivitis and arthritis (REITER's syndrome), best give MED. first even if all the rest would indicate SULPH.
- MED. mostly sleeps on the abdomen, SULPH. less so.

NATRUM MURIATICUM (NAT-M.) AND PULSATILLA (PULS.)

If you think you have a NAT-M-. or PULS.-patient in front of you, but the patient likes fat, think of SULPH.

IN WHICH ACUTE CASES DO YOU THINK OF SULPH.?

DIARRHŒA

In children if the diarrhœa smells like spoiled eggs or is very offensive, and if there is itching on anus after stool, which is aggravated by washing.

CONJUNCTIVITIS

With agglutinated eyes in the morning.

ASTHMA

In patients who are warm blooded, have a red face and who want the windows open (K. p. 770: respiration, difficult, open, wants doors and windows). They perspire and are thirsty.
The asthma is worse at night. Think of it with people working in a sulphur mine.

ERUPTIONS

All kinds of eruptions with a lot of itching. The patients scratch until the skin is bleeding. Mostly, the skin is moist and the complaints are worse after bathing.
Very often, there are eruptions round anus with a lot of itching at night.
SULPH. sometimes has big ulcers (if there is a continuous discharge of yellow pus, rather think of CALC-S.).

GASTRITIS

The stomach trouble is worse while standing (K. p. 514: stomach, pain, standing, while) and during the menses (K. p. 514: stomach, pain, menses, during).
Mostly, there is a burning sensation extending to the throat, accompanied by sour eructations.

COMMON COLD

They have a red face with very red lips (K. p. 363: discoloration, red lips). They are thirsty, perspire offensively and have to uncover their feet in an acute disease.

HEADACHE

- The most frequent SULPH.-headache is a burning feeling on the forehead and on the vertex which is ameliorated by cold applications. Mostly, the patient has a lot of perspiration in his

hair (K. p. 223: head, perspiration, occiput).
- SULPH. can get a headache by smelling eggs.
- SULPH. sometimes gets a headache by sitting in the sun.

COMPLEMENTARY REMEDIES TO SULPH.

- ACONITUM (ACON.):
    Complementary to SULPH. in acute physical problems, e.g. a common cold.

- ARSENICUM ALBUM (ARS.):
    Can form the complement to SULPH. for psychological problems with fear.

- RHUS-TOXICODENDRON (RHUS-T.):
    (must be added 3rd degree as complement to SULPH., see K. p. 1454) Especially for arthritis by getting wet. The patient is chilly and restless.

- CALCAREA. CARBONICA (CALC.).:
    When the patient was better with SULPH. and had an aversion to eggs before, while he now likes them, had a desire for fat and now an aversion, was warm blooded before and now chilly, he needs CALC. This means that the patient has evolved to a higher degree in his health. CALC. is then considered to be the strongest level of health which a patient can reach.

- PULSATILLA (PULS.)

- MERCURIUS SOLUBILIS (MERC.)

- PYROGENIUM (PYROG.):
    Here, we find a very seriously ill patient. He stinks (the smell is to be compared with a rotting dead animal). The patient shows a septic high fever. Characteristic is <u>that the pulse rate is not as you would expect</u> e.g.: <u>a very low pulse rate of 45/min. with a fever of 40°</u> (d.d. DIG.).

    PYROG. is a nosode, made of meat, rotted in the sun for a couple of weeks.
    This life threatening situation of PYROG. must be distinguished from the analogous picture of <u>BAPTISIA</u>: The patient is also seriously ill. Everything is offensive, especially the breath. The face is swollen and dark red. There is a dark line in the middle of the tongue, and sometimes the patients salivates (d.d. MERC.). BAPT. have strange delusions like:
    - their body is too large for the bed
    - only their head is in bed, the rest beside the bed
    - one leg isn't attached to the body and they are looking for it everywhere.
    (K. p. 15: confusion, intoxicated, as if; K. p. 22: delusions, body, scattered about bed, tossed about to get the pieces together).

ANTIDOTES FOR SULPH.

1st antidote = CHAMOMILE TEA

2nd antidote = FAT

PAPER CASE : SULPHUR

1st Consultation

- This case concerns a young man, 21 years old, 80 kg, height 1.97 m.
- He is very tall.
- His problem is ACNE on the face and on the back since the age of 6. The whole face is covered, except the nose and the forehead.
- His face is red and hot, and looks greasy (his hair too).
- After shaving, his skin is burning.
- The acne is aggravated by getting angry and is better in the summer at the seaside.
- The patient also suffers from stomach troubles: a burning pain with sour eructations to the mouth. The stomach trouble is aggravated by irritability and after food.
- The patient is warm blooded +++ but has cold feet.
- Mostly, he perspires on the face.
- He drinks a lot of water, he is very thirsty.
- His stool is offensive ++.
- He sleeps on his left side.
- He has a fear of high places +++.
- His appetite is normal, he likes sour ++++, green fruit +++, oranges +++, spicy +++, lemons +++ and milk ++.
- He feels happier and better at the seaside.
- He bites his nails and feels better at night than at day.

DISCUSSION BY VASSILIS

- Here, d.d. MED. - SULPH. is difficult.
- For MED. are the very strong desires, amelioration at the seaside and at night and the desire for green fruit (d.d. CALC-S.).
- Nevertheless, the patient's main problem is <u>acne, with all SULPH. signs</u> (greasy skin, red face). Besides, there is the <u>stomach trouble</u> with again real SULPH. complaints.
- Psychologically, his only problem is his <u>strong fear of heights</u>, which gives more points to SULPH.
- The patient is <u>warm blooded</u> and has an <u>offensive stool</u>, which counts in favour of SULPH.
- At the beginning, the case looks pure SULPH. up to the desires, afterwards it looks as if the therapist asked all MED. information, which gives the wrong picture.

The patient was given <u>SULPH. M.</u>

<u>1 month later</u>

During the first 14 days, the patient psychologically felt bad and irritable because of the aggravation of acne. Now, the patient feels generally better, the acne is better and the stomach troubles disappeared after 5 days.

The patient was given <u>nothing</u>.

<u>1 month later</u>

The acne is completely cured and the patient feels better from that moment on.

LIVE CASE : MAGNESIA CARBONICA

- The case concerns a 3-year-old child.
- Since he was born, the child has been crying in his sleep, he seems to have intestinal cramps. During the day, there is no problem, only, the child is sometimes irritable and may cry and stamp then.
- The child catches a cold very quickly in cold windy weather, and if so, the problems at night are worse. Then, the face is covered with perspiration.
- The child has never slept the whole night, he wakes up between 11 and 12 p.m. Sometimes, he wakes up at 6 a.m. with an urge to stool.
- In case of intestinal cramps at night, the parents must rub over the abdomen with their hands, then, the flatus comes and everything goes better afterwards.
- During the last months, there are less stomach troubles at night, but the child frequently has a cold and every 2 or 3 weeks, he has fits of coughing, especially in the day.
- He often picks his nose with a finger.
- There was a case of TB in the family. The child seldom grinds his teeth, only if he is ill.
- Sensitivity to temperature: he has warm hands and warm feet. In bed, the feet have to be uncovered. Yet, the child can't bear cold, especially cold wind.
- The child perspires little.
- He sleeps on his back.
- He drinks a lot and in large quantities.
- Food: desires sweets ++, likes honey, likes butter ++ and eggs. He has an aversion to vegetables and potatoes +++.

- He is afraid of noise, darkness, and doesn't want any water on the face.
- The child needs a lot of attention and asks many questions.
- When the child got his teeth, all the troubles were worse and there was diarrhœa.
- During the interview, the child seems very calm.

DISCUSSION BY VASSILIS

- The main problem of the child seems to have been the <u>stomach</u>, since his birth.
- <u>CHAMOMILLA</u> is the only remedy that weeps during sleep, without any reason (K. p. 94: weeping, sleep, during). CHAM. is also known for intestinal colics in babies and children. But the only thing that relieves with CHAM. is carrying the child and walking with it, and this symptom is missing here (K. p. 10: carried, desire to be).
  The child has had CHAM. a few times and only had a little amelioration.
- One of the most important remedies for abdominal cramps is <u>MAGNESIA PHOSPHORICA</u>. This remedy helps very well with abdominal cramps which are ameliorated by rubbing or putting the palm of the hand on it (by the warmth of the hand).
- On the other hand, for abdomen, pain, night, on waking, and at 1 a.m., <u>MAGNESIA MURIATICA</u> is mentioned (K. p. 556).
- The remedy with the <u>strongest aversion for vegetables</u> (K. p. 482: aversion vegetables) is <u>MAGNESIA CARBONICA</u>. MAG-C. has a strong <u>desire for butter</u> and desire bread (K. p. 484: desire bread; desire bread and butter). MAG-C. uncovers the feet at night (K. p. 1222: uncover, inclination to, feet).
- From the 3 MAGNESIA'S, Vassilis prefers here MAG-C. Most of the keynotes are for MAG-C. and this remedy is <u>complementary to</u> CHAM. (K. p. 1443 and 1449), so it will complete the effects of CHAM.
- In BOERICKE's materia medica (p. 415), we read in the modalities of MAG-C. that they <u>are aggravated by the warmth of the bed</u>, and also by <u>cold wind</u>, which is the case in this child.

- Vassilis first thought of NUX-V., afterwards of CUPR. (for the abdominal cramps) and then of the MAGNESIAS from which MAG-C. gets most confirmation. MAGNESIAS are difficult to find in homœopathy (MAG-M. is very similar to NAT-M.).

- The child is given <u>MAG-C. 200</u> for the following reasons:

    - aversion vegetables
    - desire butter
    - heat foot uncover
    - complementary to CHAM.

ALLERGIC CONDITIONS

There are several kinds of allergic conditions:

1. HAY FEVER
   - If there are only eye and nose symptoms: allergic rhinitis.
   - If there are lung symptoms: allergic asthma.

2. ALLERGIC ERUPTIONS

3. ALLERGY TO FOOD

4. ALLERGY TO ALLOPATHIC MEDICATION

In the next lecture, Vassilis will discuss **allergic rhinitis.**

REMEDIES AND THEIR CHARACTERISTIC SYMPTOMS IN ALLERGIC RHINITIS

If the constitutional remedy of a patient is clear, preferably give this for his allergy. If, however, it is a complicated case, you will often need a specific remedy in an acute attack of allergic rhinitis (in spring). In addition, when the hay fever season is over, you'll have to continue the constitutional treatment of the patient. You will find more details about this theory in a future volume "How to take the case and How to handle the patient".

ALLIUM CEPA (ALL–C.)

- It is the most frequent remedy for allergic rhinitis: 20 to 30 % of the cases (K. p. 326: nose, coryza, annual (hay fever)).
- The most characteristic symptom for ALL-C. is a discharge from nose that is caustic and burning (K. p. 331: nose, discharge, excoriating, left nostril, from) so that the nose feels hot. The top of the nose and the upper lip are red and swollen.
- The lachrymation on the contrary is not caustic or excoriating (K. p. 331: nose, discharge, excoriating, bland discharge from eyes, with; K. p. 268: eye, tears, bland).

- Mostly, there is a headache at the same time (K. p. 138: head, pain, coryza, with). The patient wants to close his eyes or he/she makes eye movements. Sometimes, they see flashes of light before the eyes.
- Mostly, there is a nasal obstruction because of oedema of the mucosa.
- ALL-C. has more allergic rhinitis in summer than in spring (K. p. 326: nose, coryza, annual (hay fever), August, in).
- They are aggravated by warmth (K. p. 329: nose, coryza, warm room) and are better outside and in open air (d.d. PULS.). If they come in afterwards, the problem may start again.
- Sometimes, the face feels warm.
- The afternoon hours are always worst.
- Be careful with someone who used to suffer from asthma and now has an allergic rhinitis. Vassilis saw the asthma come back after ALL-C. (this risk is even greater after a tonsillectomy).
- They can sneeze very often.
- They can have the sensation as if there is something sharp in the throat.
- The allergic rhinitis can start on the left and go to the right afterwards (K. p. 325: nose, coryza, left to right) (d.d. LACH.).

WYETHIA (WYE.)

- The allergy is mainly situated in nose and pharynx and shows an oedema there. The problem often starts by contact with chamomile or other flowers.
- Most characteristic is the itching on the palate or in the back of the throat (K. p. 406: mouth, itching, palate; K. p. 454: throat, itching; K. p. 340: nose, tiching, posterior nares). The itching extends to the ear. WYE. has this symptom in a common cold too. The patient tries to rub the palate with his tongue. They sometimes scratch the palate directly with a finger. To remove the itching in the ear, they can hold a finger in it, or rub the ear with a finger and, simultaneously, rub the palate with their tongue.

- There may be pain in the throat because of the oedema or because of the cough.
- If there is in addition a sensation as if the blood is rising to the head or the face, you can be sure of WYE.
- Sometimes, there is a burning sensation in the mouth.
- The patient continuously tries to clear the pharynx with a kind of continuous superficial cough or by hawking.
- With WYE., we sometimes find a headache when they perspire. If the perspiration stops, the headache will disappear.
- WYE. sometimes has chilliness at 10 or 11 p.m.

ARUM TRIPHYLLUM (ARUM-T.)

- Is frequently seen in children with hay fever or rhinitis: they have numbness or itching on the lips and nose (K. p. 379: face, itching, lips; K. p. 339: nose, itching). They constantly pick or scratch their lips or pick their nose (K. p. 348: nose, picking nose; picking nose until it bleeds; K. p. 391: face, picking, lips). Sometimes, they take some mucus out of their nose.
- They have a sensation as if their lips are itching from the inside; sometimes, even their gums are itching.
- They continuously wet their lips with the tongue, scratch their lips with their teeth or suck on them.
- The lips are red, excoriated or cracked (K. p. 357: face, cracked lips). The lips often bleed because of the constant itching or picking (K. p. 355: bleeding lips).
- Even around the lips and on the chin, the skin can be irritated, excoriated or cracked. This is because they continuously scratch their lips with their teeth.
  In a chronic case, we see a child with a line above and below the lips because of the chronic scratching with the teeth over the lips.
- Think of ARUM-T. in a child with allergic rhinitis and cracks in the corners of the mouth (K. p. 326: nose, coryza, annual; K. p. 357: cracks, corners of mouth).
- On blowing the nose, there can be discharge of bloody and stringy nasal mucus.

- The complaints are mostly on the left side: the left nostril and the left eye (K. p. 325: nose, coryza, left).
- In ARUM-T., usually we don't find an allergic asthma or dyspnoea. The most characteristic symptom is the <u>itching on the lips and in the nose</u>, often combined with nasal obstruction.

EUPHRASIA (EUPHR.)

- Here, we find the opposite of ALL-C.: <u>the tears are caustic </u>(K. p. 267: eye, tear, acrid; tears burning) while <u>the discharge from the nose is not caustic</u> or excoriating (K. p. 329: nose, discharge, blandy).
- With EUPHR., <u>the itching is worst in the eyes</u>. There is a thick discharge from the eyes. Sometimes, there is a swelling round the eyes. The eye symptoms are worse in warm wind (K. p. 246: eye, lachrymation, wind, in) and in the morning. They can have very red conjunctiva, and the eyes are very often stuck up in the morning.
- In the morning, the patient can feel mucus in the trachea. They try very hard to hawk up the mucus until they have to vomit (sometimes, the whole breakfast is thrown up).

- D.d. <u>SULPH.</u>: They have the feeling that there is sand in the eyes and they continuously try to rub it out. SULPH. has offensive discharges.

- D.d. <u>PULS.</u>: Is also aggravated by warm wind. If you have all EUPHR.-symptoms, and the only thing that ameliorates is cold water in the face, you must think of PULS.

SABADILLA (SABAD.)

- The most characteristic symptom of SABAD. is the spasmodic, repetitive sneezing more than 10 times one after another (K. p. 351: nose, sneezing, paroxysmal). If the patient is driving a car at that moment, he'll have to stop to finish his sneezing.
- There is lachrymation from the eyes, the eyelids are burning and red. The face is warm.
- The nose is obstructed and yet there can be a discharge.
- The complaints are worse in the open air and better in the warm wind (contrary to EUPHR.).
- The complaints are aggravated by flowers and can start with the smell of flowers, especially in the spring.
- SABAD. often has an aversion to onions (K. p. 482: aversion onions), at other times they desire onions.

SINAPIS NIGRA (SIN-N.)

- Here, the sneezing is worst at night, during the KALI-hours (K. p. 350: nose, sneezing, night, lying down, while). The nasal obstruction too is worst at night.

ARUNDO (ARUND.)

- According to the experience of Vassilis, it works very seldom. Rather give all other possible remedies before you give ARUND.

AILANTUS GLANDULOSA (AIL.)

- Here, the characteristic symptom is the serious nasal obstruction which makes the patient sad. They have the feeling that they can't breath anymore because of the nasal obstruction, although the nasal obstruction itself doesn't seem very serious.
- The nose is troubling them terribly. They have the feeling as if there is a wound in the nose. They sometimes complain about pain in the left nostril.
- It is a rare remedy which you might need only once or twice in your life.

TEUCRIUM (TEUCR.)

- Here, the reason for the nasal obstruction is mostly a nasal polyp (K. p. 349: nose, polypus). The polyp doesn't have to be on the right side as mentioned in the books, it can also be on the left side.
- The patient has a sensation as if there are ants in his nose (K. p. 338: nose, formication, root).
- The nose is obstructed (K. p. 340: nose, obstruction, right) and there is a dirty, offensive discharge. The trouble is worse in damp weather and is aggravated by the warmth of the bed.
- They sometimes get a sinusitis with the symptoms of KALI-BI., because of the mechanical obstruction of the nasal polyp.

STICTA PULMONARIA (STICT.)

- If the only symptom is: a very strong sensation of nasal obstruction , without discharge.
- The patient feels the nasal obstruction at the root of the nose (like KALI-BI.) (K. p. 341: nose, obstruction, root, at). The nose feels dry.

- The patient is constantly blowing his nose without result (K. p. 335: nose, dryness, blowing nose, compelled, but no discharge). If the patient is able to get out a little nasal mucus, he'll feel much better.
- Sometimes, they have a headache.

LEMNA MINOR (LEM–M.)

- If nothing else helps and a <u>nasal obstruction</u> is the only symptom, you can think of LEM-M.
- Vassilis has given it twice in his life with succes.

LIVE CASE : CALCAREA CARBONICA

<u>1st consultation</u>

- The case concerns a woman of 34 years. She has 3 children.
- The patient has been very tired, ill and sick for her whole life. She wants to be alone, left in peace. In a crowd, she is irritable.
- Her eyes are tired, she has a headache, and sometimes, she is dizzy. She can't think when she is tired, she wants to be alone with her thoughts.
- She is easily chilly, has cold hands and feet, wears socks in bed.
- She falls asleep on her right side.
- If she is on a high place, she has a feeling as if she will die.
- She is afraid if her husband comes home late, she always fears the worst.
- She doesn't like the sun, she feels sick then.
- She doesn't like to swim.
- She is afraid of all animals, in an elevator, in a narrow street or in a crowd. She doesn't like sleeping in complete darkness. In the dark, she sometimes has the feeling as if someone is behind her.
- When everything goes wrong, she sometimes thinks she's going crazy.
- Stool is normal.
- Her nails break easily.

DISCUSSION BY VASSILIS

This is a clear example of CALC.
The patient displays nearly all the characteristic information we need for CALC. For this reason, Vassilis gives us the essential information of CALC.

ESSENTIAL INFORMATION FOR CALCAREA CARBONICA

- They are weak, especially while going upstairs and downstairs (K. p. 1345: ascending agg.) or while walking fast. This makes them short of breath (K. p. 768: respiration, difficult, ascending).

- They are chilly. Their feet are coldest when they go to bed, that's why they wear socks to go to sleep and either they wear them during the whole night or they have to take them off after a few hours because their feet are too warm then (K. p. 963: extremities, coldness, foot, night, bed, in).
  In the summer, they sometimes can't bear the sun.

- They are often afraid of going mad, especially when their mind is weakened (K. p. 45: fear, insanity, of). This symptom prevails over all the other symptoms! and must lead us directly to CALC. or PULS.

- CALC. has more fears than any other remedy:
    - bad dreams and nightmares
    - fear of high places and dizziness when on a high place (K. p. 100: vertigo, high places)
    - fear of narrow places (K. p. 46: fear, narrow places: here, CALC. may be added 2nd degree)
    - afraid in the dark (K. p. 43: fear, dark)
    - afraid of water and afraid to swim in the sea
    - afraid that someone is behind them in the dark (K. p. 30: delusion, people, sees, behind him, someone is)
    - afraid of getting ill (K. p. 7: anxiety, health, about; K. p. 44: fear, disease, of impending)

- afraid of death (K. p. 44: fear, death, of)
- afraid of thunderstorms (K. p. 47: fear, thunderstorm, of: may be added 2nd degree)
- afraid of animals (K. p. 43: fear, animals, of: may be added 3rd degree); they are especially afraid of insects, mice and spiders.

- CALC. mostly develops constipation (here, this symptom is missing) (K. p. 11: cheerful, constipated, when).

- The nails are fragile and break easily (K. p. 954: extremities, brittle finger nails).

- They often look on the dark side of life.

- They are often obese and plump (K. p. 1376: obesity).

- Don't forget that CALC. can also be slender and without any fears.

CONCLUSION

If it was about a warm-blooded person, we had to give PULS. because of the fear of insanity.
Now, it is clearly a CALC.-case. She is a healthy person with a good prognosis.

The patient is given CALC. M.

LIVE CASE : GRAPHITES

<u>1st consultation</u>

- The case concerns a 5-year-old girl with <u>skin problems for some years</u> and recently also <u>bronchitis attacks every month.</u>
- She has cracks behind the ears, but especially eruptions on legs and in the hollows of the knee.
  She has serious itching, especially at night. The itching is worse after bathing, when she gets warm and when she is angry. The skin problems have been better since she stopped fat and milk in her food.
- When she has an attack of <u>bronchitis</u>, she coughs at night, which wakes her every hour, particularly between 10 p.m. and 3 a.m.
- She is warm blooded, feels warm in bed but doesn't perspire.
- She likes to eat: bread +++, milk, eggs, cheese, meat and chocolate.
- She is not very thirsty.
- She sometimes walks barefooted.
- Her character: she is sweet, active, knows what she wants. She is not a mummy's child.

DISCUSSION BY VASSILIS

- With children having <u>cracks behind the ears</u>, you have to think of GRAPH. first (K. p. 288: ear, eruptions behind ears, cracks) Eruptions and cracks in the hollows of the knee are also characteristic of GRAPH. (K. p. 970: extremities, cracks, skin, joints, bends of; K. p. 1001: extremities, eruption, knee, hollow of).
- We can take the following rubrics for the problem of bronchitis:
    - K. p. 764: asthma, after midnight
    - K. p. 767: difficult respiration, night, in bed

    If asthma was the main problem, we had to give ARS.
- In Boericke p. 311 and 312, we read in GRAPH. "modalities" that there is an aggravation at night, in warmth, and in "respiratory" is mentioned that there may be chronic hoarseness with skin affections.
- Because the skin is the main problem here and because GRAPH. covers skin as well as lung problems, Vassilis starts in this case with GRAPH.

    We do not find here the typical moist eczema with the glutinous honey-yellow discharge (K. p. 1311: skin, eruptions, discharging, glutinous).
- A remedy you might also think of is KALI-IODATUM, because the worst troubles occur after midnight (worst hours 2 a.m. - 4 a.m.), the aggravation of skin eruptions by warmth, and the amelioration in open air and cold (like PULS.).

CONCLUSION

The child is given <u>GRAPH. 200</u>.

REMEDIES AND THEIR CHARACTERISTIC SYMPTOMS IN SKIN DISORDERS

GRAPHITES (GRAPH.)

- The eruptions of GRAPH. can be found over the whole body, but especially in the neck, round and behind the ears (K. p. 288: ear, eruption, behind ears, cracks), on the hands, on the legs and in the hollow of the knee (K. p. 970: extremities, cracks, skin, joints, bends of; K. p. 1001: extremities, eruption, knee, hollow of).
- The eruptions are mostly moist and there is a glutinous honey-yellow discharge (K. p. 1311: skin, eruptions, discharging, glutinous; discharging yellow). In case of acne on the face with yellow discharge, we rather think of CALC-S.
- The discharge from the skin is sometimes offensive. The perspiration is mostly offensive (K. p. 1298: perspiration, odor, offensive).
- They mostly have brittle finger nails (K. p. 954: extremities, brittle finger nails) or crippled nails (K. p. 978: crippled finger nails; crippled toe nails) and sometimes nails like lime (K. p. 1207: thick nails).
- If someone suffers from asthma, and is ameliorated by eating, you have to think of GRAPH. (K. p. 764: respiration, asthmatic, eating amel.).
- With GRAPH., you will often find an aversion to fish, sweets and salt (K. p. 480: stomach, aversion, fish; K. p. 482: aversion, sweets; aversion salt food).

- GRAPH. easily weeps from music (K. p. 94: weeping, music, from).

PETROLEUM (PETR.)

- Characteristic is the <u>dryness</u> (K. p. 1308: skin, dry) and the <u>cracks in the skin</u> (K. p. 1305: skin, cracks).
- The skin problems are clearly worse in the winter (K. p. 1305: skin, cracks, winter) and better in the summer.
- PETR. has an aversion to fat (K. p. 480: stomach, aversion, fats and rich food). When there is a desire for fat, rather think of NIT-AC.
- In case of dryness of the palms of the hands and bleeding cracks (K. p. 970: extremities, cracks, hands, deep and bleeding), think of PETR. in the first place, of NIT-AC. in the second and of SARS. in the third place.

RHUS VENENATA (RHUS-V.)

- We find very small vesicles filled with a watery fluid, especially on the hands and genitalia (K. p; 696: genitalia, eruptions).
- The only thing that relieves the serious itching is <u>hot water</u>.
- Other remedies for skin diseases which are ameliorated by warm applications are RHUS-T. and ARS.

RHUS TOXICODENDRON (RHUS-T.)

- The patient mostly suffers from arthritis or stiffness in the fingers.

LACHESIS (LACH.)

- Here, you will find little tumours in the skin. Between them, you can find <u>dark or blue spots</u> on the face.
- The face is very red or bluish.
- Old scars in LACH. show a blue colour just as old scars in SIL. show a hole. Except for the blue discoloration, the skin remains intact.

CALCAREA SULPHURICA (CALC-S.)

- Here, we see wounds in the skin with spontaneous <u>yellow discharge</u> or where the yellow pus can be pressed out.
- CALC-S. is mostly warm blooded.

HEPAR SULPHURIS (HEP.)

- Here, you see the same wounds with the yellow discharge as in CALC-S.
- You can also find crypts in the skin where you can press out yellow pus.
- HEP. is very chilly, contrary to CALC-S.

PAPER CASE : OLEANDER

1st consultation 1980

- The case concerns a child, 7 years old, 20 kg.
- He has had an allergic dermatitis for 4 years. It started with recurring conjunctivitis which was accompanied by oedema, redness and swellings round the eyes. Afterwards, it extended to the whole face, the hands and the feet. After treatment with steroid ointments, only the eruptions round the eyes remained. The dermatologists said there was no treatment for this problem, the case was incurable according to them. They predicted it would disappear spontaneously at the age of 20.
- Now, there are serious eruptions round the eyes and the mouth. We see small ulcerations. There is a swelling round the eyes.
- There is a lot of itching +++, especially in bed, in damp weather ++ and while perspiring. The hands and feet are itching too when going to sleep.
- There is constipation with hard stool.
- The child mainly perspires on the neck.
- He is warm blooded.
- The child sleeps on the left side.
- He is closed, has few friends, is very sensitive, sympathetic ++, anxious ++, restless++.
- This child never sits quietly, always walks around and is irritable.
- He likes ice cream ++, fat ++++, pasta++, olives ++, oranges ++, but they are not given to the child because they aggravate the eruptions.

- Skin problems which are aggravated by ORANGES, CITRUS FRUITS, LEMONS OR ACIDS are very characteristic of OLEANDER (must be added 3rd degree on K. p. 1363: food, oranges agg.; and in Boericke). It is strange that most OLND.-patients crave for oranges.

- The skin problems are mostly situated on the head. It is an eruption which is difficult to treat. Sometimes, the hairs will break off in a circle.

- They can also have herpes after having eaten a lot of acids. With tourists on holiday in southern countries, who eat a lot of citrus fruits and suddenly have eruptions or herpes, we must think of OLND.

- OLND. is generally aggravated by undressing (K. p. 1410: undressing, after, agg.), i.e. mostly when they go to bed.

- The itching of OLND. is aggravated by undressing (K. p. 1329: skin, itching, undressing, agg.), at night in bed, and after eating oranges.

CONCLUSION

The patient was given OLEANDER M.

Very soon after the remedy, the child changed completely. Before, it didn't want to go to school anymore because of the bad appearance: other children didn't want to play with the patient. After the remedy, the child wanted to go to school again and the eruptions disappeared progressively and rather quickly. With this one dose, the child hasn't had any problems for 7 years now.

PAPER CASE : OLEANDER

1st consultation

- The case concerns a 9-year-old girl.
- She has had eczema round the right eye, round the mouth and on the right side of the face for 3 years. She has also had it round the left eye since she was treated with steroid ointment.
- There are also eruptions in the hollow of the knee and on the elbows.
- The complaints are worse in the spring and better at the seaside +.
- Tomatoes +++ and oranges +++ aggravate her seriously.
- She scratches until it is bleeding.
- She is very sensitive, has a lot of fears, is irritable.
- She studies well, has an open character.
- She sleeps on her right side.
- She likes pasta, chocolate, ice cream, chips.
- She is very thirsty.

DISCUSSION BY VASSILIS

- In general, we get a lot of information indicating PHOS.
- Because of the serious aggravation by tomatoes and oranges, we have to give OLEANDER first, this remedy prevails.

CONCLUSION

The patient was given OLEANDER.

The eczema disappeared completely. Later, PHOS. was needed for another problem and she was better immediatly.

PAPER CASE : APIS

1st consultation

- The case concerns a women of 32 years, 50 kg., 1.62 m.
- 3 months ago, she had a cholecystogram and she had a general allergic reaction. She has been swollen completely and has had a burning sensation on her arms and legs since. In the morning and evening, there is itching too. She feels better with cold applications and when there is a cold wind or air blowing.
- She is very warm blooded and uncovers her feet at night.
- She has suffered from swellings of the ankles, worst in the evening between 9 and 10 p.m., for several years.
- She is a little thirsty, likes to drink ice water +++.
- She can't sleep very well when she is angry, she often wakes up at 3 a.m., can't fall asleep except on the right side.
- She is very irritable ++++, she weeps easily, sighs +++.
- With serious itching, she is hysterical and short of breath.
- She is afraid to go to sleep alone at night, afraid of thunder storms, worried about her childres, has a fear of high places.
- She doesn't feel well in the afternoon but is better in the evening.
- Sexually normal.
- She is closed and easily angry.
- She desires sweets +++, refreshing things ++, sour.
- She doesn't like fruit.
- She has an aversion to milk +++ and fat +++.

- Since she has had this allergy, she has been suffering from headaches at about 10 - 11 a.m.
- If she takes an aspirin, her face will swell.

DISCUSSION BY VASSILIS

- In case of a chronic swelling of the ankles, think first of MED., then of APIS. (K. p. 1201: extremities, swelling, ankle).
- We get a lot of information indicating NAT-M. in this case:
  She is introverted and closed, a headache at 10 a.m., aversion to fat and milk, fear of heights, afraid of thunder storms, warm blooded.
- She has shown the picture of APIS. since she had the cholecystogram. She suffers from an allergic dermatitis with a burning sensation and swellings everywhere. Cold applications and cold wind ameliorate everything. She is very irritable ++ (APIS. can be more irritable than NUX-V.).
- It is possible that APIS. is a new level which has been put on a NAT-M.-constitution, or the APIS.-symptoms have become clear since the cholecystogram. But the patient has suffered from swollen ankles for several years and this argues for the second possibility.

GENERAL INFORMATION ABOUT APIS.

- APIS. has swellings which look as if they will burst.

- APIS. can never be chilly (SULPH. PULS. and NAT-M. can be chilly exceptionally).

- APIS. can have a headache at 10 a.m. or from 10 a.m. to 6 p.m. (K. p. 134: head, pain, forenoon, 10 a.m.; 10 a.m. to 6 p.m.).

- APIS. is complementary to NAT-M., therefore, some symptoms are equal.

- APIS. is mentioned on K. p. 769: respiration, difficult, eruptive diseases, with; K. p. 771: respiration, difficult, suppressed eruptions, from. You will only find this symptom in an acute situation, not in a chronic situation. Perhaps, the concrete situation where this symptom will occur is:
  - eruptions and swelling in the neck, the face and the uvula which causes dyspnoea.
  - a bee sting round the mouth which produces oedema of the larynx and causes dyspnoea with danger of suffocation.

- After a bee sting with general symptoms, you'd better give APIS. 200. In case of a serious allergic reaction, you'd better give APIS. M.

- APIS. can have an allergy to quite a lot of things.

CONCLUSION

The patient was given APIS. M. After 5 days, all skin problems had disappeared, she became calm and has been well until now.

PAPER CASE : HELLEBORUS NIGER

<u>1st consultation</u>

- The case concerns a man, 55 years old, who has had a serious <u>memory problem</u> for 4 years. He can remember almost nothing. Six years ago, he had an operation for <u>lung cancer</u>, and some time later, his memory problem started.
- He forgets everything, doesn't remember where he put things, his orientation and concentration are gone. He doesn't even know exactly how old he is. At the table, he sometimes doesn't know his place, he loses his way in a city. He does know where he lives and near his house, he won't lose his way.
- He remembers things in the remote past, but not the recent facts. E.g. if he watches television and he sees a goal, he will forget it 5 minutes later. If he talks, he can't remember afterwards what he said.
- This man is very depressed because there is nothing he can do anymore. He stopped working, can't drive anymore and what's more, he has become <u>impotent</u> during the last year. He has the feeling that he has lost everything, he'd rather be dead.
- He used to lead a very active and busy life, but he has totally changed now, says his wife. He sits all day, and at best he'll work a bit in the garden. He used to have a good memory.
- The patient sighs often, especially if he has to do something.
- He can't bear his wife telling him what to do.
- He preferably sleeps on his left side.
- He has become very chilly since his illness. In bed, he uses an electric blanket.
- He is very thirsty for cold water, cold milk ++, at night he likes

beer. He desires salt and dislikes sweets ++.

DISCUSSION BY VASSILIS

- This patient is very ill on his deepest mental level. He used to have lung cancer (ill on physical level). Since his lung cancer was removed, the centre of his illness has moved to a much deeper level and from that moment on, his recent memory has failed.
- The patient is 55 years old and looks as if he is 70. Here, we have to think of remedies giving a strong weakening of the memory: the top 3 of these are: 1. PIC-AC., 2. HELL. and 3. ANAC.
- If there was a destruction of cerebral cells or a disturbance in the metabolism of the cerebral cells, the top 4 would be as follows in hierarchical order: 1. HELL., 2. PLB., 3. ZINC., 4. CAUST.
- In this case, it's no use starting from the remedies who sigh a lot or who are impotent, this is not the patient's main problem and if you would give a remedy for impotence, it could be possible that you would have opened the sexual channel to lose even more cerebral energy.

THE MOST IMPORTANT REMEDIES IN CASE OF AN AFFECTION OF THE CEREBRAL CELLS

1. HELLEBORUS NIGER (HELL.): see further.

2. PLUMBUM (PLB.):
   mostly shows trembling (as in Parkinson's disease) and extreme physical fatigue (K. p. 1212: extremities, trembling, hand, holding objects, on).

3. ZINCUM METALLICUM (ZINC.) :
   weakness in the spinal column and in the legs with restless feet (K. p. 1188: restlessness, feet, sitting, while).

4. CAUSTICUM (CAUST.):

shows paralysis, caused by affection of cerebral cells (K. p. 1390: paralysis, gradually appearing).

THE MOST IMPORTANT REMEDIES IN CASE OF A WEAKNESS OF MEMORY

1. PICRICUM ACIDUM (PIC-AC.):

can do physical work very well from the morning to the evening, but the slightest mental effort will give exhaustion. They develop a real aversion to books (K. p. 41: exertion, agg., from mental).

2. HELLEBORUS (HELL.): see further

3. ANACARDIUM (ANAC.):

There is a lack of self-confidence (K. p. 13: confidence, want of self). They think they are worthless, that their parents or teachers don't believe in them and that's why they use all their energy to study, to prove they really can do something. They use so much energy that they may suddenly collapse: they won't remember anything, they can't pass their exams. They get angry and start swearing (K. p. 17: cursing).

GENERAL INFORMATION ABOUT HELLEBORUS NIGER (HELL.)

- The weakness of memory is not caused by bad circulation in the cerebral cells, but by a kind of encephalitis in a certain place in the brain. It is mostly seen in cancer patients, in meningitis, or in old people.

- The main symptom is the <u>weakness of memory</u> (K. p. 65: memory, weakness of; say for what is about to). They are better in the morning, the worst time is in the afternoon from 2, 3 or 4 p.m. to 8 p.m. (K. p. 1342: afternoon 4 p.m. to 8 p.m.; d.d. LYC.). During these aggravation hours, they are mostly sad too.

- They sigh without knowing it (see Boericke p. 321 "mind").

- They look sympathetic: they know they are weak and need help and affection of others. They are afraid to do something wrong. They resemble PHOS.: the family says they have become very kind and sweet since their weakness of memory.

- Sometimes, they forget their name or address. They can lose the way to their own house.

- This remedy can also be used in case of hydrocephaly (see Boericke).

CONCLUSION

- The best remedy to start with is <u>HELL.</u> It is possible that with this remedy the memory will improve and the earlier lung problem will come back. If the lung will be treated allopathicly, the memory problems may start again. It is a difficult case with an uncertain prognosis.

- The patient is given <u>HELL. 200.</u>

REMEDIES AND THEIR CHARACTERISTIC SYMPTOMS IN CANCER

Vassilis indicates when a case should be suspected of having cancer and how you should handle a cancer patient. Besides, he warns us only to take cancer patients in well-chosen situations.
You will find more information about this subject in future volumes.

CONIUM (CON.)

The central idea with CONIUM is:

INDURATION

This sclerosis or hardening can be found on every level:

- Mentally, they show fixed ideas.
- Physically, they show tumours.

- If a CONIUM-patient develops a tumour somewhere, it is always suspected to be malignant (K. p. 693: genitalia, cancer). Tumours with a SIL.-picture are more likely to be benign.

- CONIUM is mostly the result of <u>suppression of sexual energy</u> (K. p. 1399: sexual, desire, suppression of, agg.). Especially a sudden unexpected break off of a sexual relationship for a long period.
  E.g.: a 50 year old man who has suddenly lost his wife and who develops prostate problems after 6 months or 1 year: Here, do think of cancer. don't give this person IGN., he needs CONIUM! With CON., you may preserve the patient in such a case from prostate cancer.
  E.g.: A religious person in the convent (a nun with cervical cancer).
  E.g.: someone who can't have coitus anymore because of a tumour in the spine and is now developing a prostate problem.

- <u>With CON., we find a lot of prostate complaints</u> (K. p. 667: prostate, gland, hardness).
    - They have to urinate frequently.
    - They have pain while urinating.
    - There is a burning pain after urination.
    - There is a pressing pain on the perineum (K. p. 634: rectum, weight, perineum).
    - At night, the patient has to get up several times to urinate.
    - The patient doesn't have a good stream while urinating and sometimes urinates on his shoes.

- <u>In CON., we find the following tumours (esp. genital tumours)</u>

    - In men: - testicular tumours
              - bladder tumours
              - prostate gland tumours
              - lung cancer

    - In women: - breast tumours
                 - uterine tumours
                 - ovarian tumours

- CON. may not be repeated too quickly, certainly not daily in 12 CH.

NATRUM MURIATICUM (NAT-M.)

Vassilis had a 15-year-old boy with the following complaint: bed-wetting with a clear picture of NAT-M. : <u>he ate salt with a spoon</u> (K. p. 486: stomach, desires salt). He gave NAT-M. 200 without any reaction. NAT-M. M. didn't cause a reaction either, the same for NAT-M 10 M. To be certain, he repeated NAT-M. 200, M. and 10 M. together from another pharmacy. He was surprised that the remedy was so clear and that there wasn't the slightest reaction, so he sent the patient to a urologist, who found polycystic kidneys on both sides. This is an organic problem that can't be ameliorated and from which the boy might die.

Always send the patient for examination when a clearly indicated remedy doesn't work, or always works shorter and shorter: such situations may indicate a serious complaint or cancer!

NUX VOMICA (NUX-V.)

Vassilis treated a patient who came for recurrent cystitis. He had several courses of treatment with antibiotics in a year, but recently they didn't help anymore.
The homœopathic history gave a clear picture of NUX-V. The patient was given NUX-V. 200, which ameliorated him spectacularly, but then he fell back. Then, the patient was given NUX-V.12 CH. daily for 30 days which ameliorated him for 1 month and then he fell back.
Vassilis gave NUX-V. M.: he was better for 5 days and fell back again always with the same picture of high fever and serious weakness. Then, Vassilis sent the patient for examination. On the chest XRay, a big tumour was found in the right lung with metastasis in the bones. The patient was then treated palliatively with homœopathy, he didn't have to take any allopathic medication and died quietly and with a clear mind.

SIL. develops especially tumours after suppression of perspiration (K. p. 1302: perspiration, suppressed, complaints from).
E.g. a protracted use of boric acid ... lead to cerebral tumour. The tumour can be benign (K. p. 277: dim... suppressed foot-sweat after).
E.g. A protracted use of armpit deodorants can lead to breast tumours in women (mostly not malignant) or to very painful but harmless armpit tumours: hydradenitis.

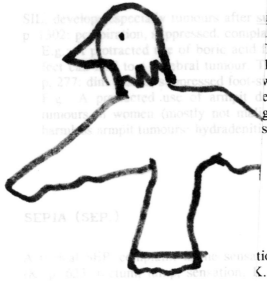

SEPIA (SEP.)

A typical SEP. complaint is the sensation of a ball or lump in anus (K. p. 667: rectum, lump sensation; K. p. 667: prostate gland, ball, sensation on sitting on it. If SEPIA doesn't help, or only helps temporarily and then the patient comes back, think of rectal cancer and have the patient examined.
Patients with this complaint (men as well as women) are often helped well and definitely with SEPIA. Possibly, we protect them without making the correct diagnosis of rectal cancer.

NITRICUM ACIDUM (NIT-AC.)

Their whole life is dominated by cancer, they run from one specialist to another until someone will find THEIR CANCER (K. p. 7: anxiety, health, about).
Vassilis had a patient whose fears were better on NIT-AC., but she dreamed she had cancer in the rectum. In order to set her mind at rest, he had her examined, but she actually had a rectal cancer (K. p. 606: rectum cancer).

NATRUM SULPHURICUM (NAT-S.)

They easily show intestinal cancer like NIT-AC. Nevertheless, the localisation of the cancer of NAT-S. is more frequently in the sigmoid and of NIT-AC. in the rectum.

AURUM MURIATICUM NATRONATUM (AUR-M-N.)

Think of it in case of uterine cancer. Mostly, it is about incurable cases of uterine carcinoma with metastasis.
When you have the picture of AUR. combined with uterine problems, think of AUR-M-N.

ABROTANUM (ABROT.)

With incurable cases of uterine cancer with metastasis, think of AB-ROT.

This is the remedy of METASTASIS. Mostly, there is an alternation between pain in the joints and diarrhœa or anal loss of blood.

E.g.: - pain in the joints or bones which is relieved when the patient has diarrhœa (K. p. 1046: extremities, pain, rheumatic, diarrhœa checked).
- the joint-complaints are worse with constipation.
- the joint-complaints are better with anal loss of blood
- with chronic or acute haemorrhoids: when they are bleeding, the pain in the joints is relieved. (K. p. 1046: extremities, pain, rheumatic, alternating with haemorrhoids).

1st consultation

- The case concerns a 30-year-old woman.
- Her main complaint has been an <u>allergic rhinitis</u> for 3 years. She has a running nose and itching eyes, sneezing, nasal obstruction. She has an itching feeling at the root of the nose.
- The allergy is worst when it is warm outside (not inside). It is better in fresh, open air. She has a lot of troubles from the moment she wakes up in the morning. It is better in rainy weather.
- She has also an <u>allergy to fruit</u>. She can only eat oranges and bananas. She has to sneeze and cough when she eats apples and peaches, it makes her mouth feel painful.
- Animals don't give her any trouble.
- <u>10 years ago, she had a stomach ULCER.</u>
- As a child, she was very closed, kept everything inside. She was easily influenced and uncertain. Now, she has been more open since her last relationship.
- She likes her work very much, but is looking for a job with more responsibilities. She likes business and management. She does her work very conscientiously.
- She lives alone.
- She only weeps when she is angry.
- She has a fear of high places, and is afraid in closed rooms because she was locked up once.
- Before the menses, she is irritable, clumsy and weeps more easily. As soon as the menses break through, it is over.

- She can't bear tight clothes.
- She sleeps on the left or right side, never on her back.
- She is chilly, always has cold hands. She likes the sun when she hasn't got an allergy.
- She has little thirst, likes orange juice, beer, wine and campari (bitter).
- She likes fish and liver. She doesn't eat the fat of meat.
- She likes spicy, sour food and boiled or fried eggs.
- Her nails are good.
- Her boyfriend had had a relationship with another woman for one year and yet she stayed with him. Then, she ended the relationship after he had told her that his other girlfriend was more important than her.
- She is rather tidy: she makes her bed in the morning after getting up.

DISCUSSION BY VASSILIS

This patient has 3 problems:

- firstly: an allergic rhinitis
- secondly: an emotional problem
- thirdly: a former ulcer

According to Vassilis, this ulcer is the centre of the case. To produce an ulcer in such a young woman, she must be a very energetic person with insufficient possibilities to express herself. The tendency to ulcers remains with this woman, because she is not satisfied with her current job and her relationship (for one year, she had stayed with the man she loved but he had another girlfriend). She has to be full of energy and emotions, but she can't use them in a healthy way.

CHARACTERISTIC INFORMATION OF NUX-V.

- She has a lot of ambition. She is not satisfied with her current job. She wants to change to do something better and to take more responsibility. NUX-V. is the remedy with most ambition, they are not easily pleased, always want to better themselves and want to climb up to a higher position.

- At an early age, she had an ulcer. She has always worked hard and wants to work even harder. NUX-V. is one of the most important remedies for a stomach ulcer because of too much ambition and because they want to work too much (K. p. 531: stomach, ulcers).

- She still thinks of her work when she is at home (NUX-V. dreams of his work: K. p. 1236: sleep, dreams, business, of).

- She thinks the opinion of others is right when they criticize her, even if she is sure about her opinion.

- She can easily get angry. NUX-V. is easily angry (K. p. 69: offended, easily).

- She works perfectly and conscientiously. In the morning, her bed must be made. NUX-V. want order round them, they are fastidious, their mind works better in an orderly evironment(K. p. 42: fastidious).

- She is irritable before the menses (K. p. 59: irritability, menses, before), weeps sometimes then. NUX-V. can be anxious before the menses (K. p. 7: anxiety, menses, before).

- She never wears tight clothes, which is typical of NUX-V. (K. p. 1348: clothing, intolerance of).

- She is chilly. NUX-V. is chilly.

- Her allergic rhinitis corresponds to the NUX-V.-picture.

  - Her running nose is better in open air (K. p. 326: nose, coryza, air, open, amel.).
  - She sneezes in the morning in bed and after getting up (K. p. 350: nose, sneezing, morning, bed, in; morning, rising, after).
  - She is better in wet weather (K. p. 1357: dry weather agg.) (d.d. CAUST.).

The patient also shows some LACH.-characteristics

- The allergy is worst in the spring (K. p. 1403: spring, in) and in the autumn (K. p. 1345: autumn agg., in).
- She can't bear tight clothes.
- There is an aggravation before the menses, and as soon as the bleeding starts, all the complaints disappear.
- She likes alcoholic drinks.
- She is aggravated by warmth.
- Nevertheless, LACH. is not possible because:
  - A LACH.-woman would never allow her boyfriend to have another girlfriend, she is too jealous for that K. p. 60: jealousy).
  - LACH. is too tired in the morning to make her bed (K. p. 1255: sleep, unrefreshing).
  - The patient is not afraid of snakes.
  - She can be in the sun if she has no allergy.

CONCLUSION

The differential diagnosis between LACH. and NUX-V. is not always easy. In this case, it is a rather clear picture of NUX-V.

The patient is given NUX-V. M.

You will find the most violent headaches in BELL. and GELS. The patients may feel they will become insane from the pain (K. p. 142: head, pain, maddening pains).

BELLADONNA-headache

- The <u>face is red and hot</u> (K. p. 362: face, discoloration, red face, headache, during).
- The <u>extremities are cold or icecold</u> (hands and feet) while they have a burning sensation in their head (K. p. 122: head, heat, coldness, extremities, with)..
- They have a sensation as if all their blood is rising to their head (K. p. 111: head, congestion, redness of face, with).
- The pupils are wide-open (K. p. 263: eye, pupils, dilated). That's why there is a strong <u>photophobia</u> (K. p. 261: eye, photophobia).
- They are better when they lie down in a dark room (K. p. 142: head, pain, lying in a dark room amel.; BELL. has this stronger than SIL.).

GELSEMIUM-headache

- The pain starts from the neck and extends all over the head (K. p. 901: back, pain, cervical region, extending, head, to, all over). With SIL., the pain starts from the neck too, but extends to the eyes (K. p. 901: back, pain, cervical region, extending, eye, to).
- The eyelids are very heavy and it is difficult to keep them open (K. p. 241: eye, heaviness, eyelids).
- The vision is blurred during the headache (K. p. 276: vision, dim, headache, during).
- They have to urinate abundantly and this relieves the headache (K. p. 150: head, pain, urination, profuse, amel.).

IRIS VERSICOLOR-headache

- Most characteristic is the diminution of vision before the headache begins (K. p. 276: vision, dim, headache, before; K. p. 166: head, pain, side, right, blurred vision before the attack).

NATRUM MURIATICUM-headache

- It is a hammering headache (K. p. 140: head, pain, hammering, morning).
- The headache starts in the morning when rising, is worst about 10 or 11 a.m. to 3 to 4 p.m. Then, the headache is better and it comes back from 5 p.m. (K. p. 134: head, pain, 10 a.m.; 10 a.m. to 3 p.m.).
- The headache is mostly on the right side.
- The headache is worse in the sun (K. p. 149: head, pain, sun, from exposure to; K. p. 1404: sun, from exposure to).

- The headache is aggravated by grief or emotional excitement (K. p. 139: head, pain, excitement of the emotions, after; K. p. 140: head, pain, grief, from; K. p. 150: head, pain, vexation, after).

SANGUINARIA-headache

- This is a frequently occuring headache-remedy, sometimes more than BELL.
- The pain starts in the right shoulder (K. p. 1052: extremities, pain, shoulder, right) or right in the neck and extends from behind the right ear upwards, or more typically to above the right eye (K. p. 159: head, pain, forehead, eyes, above right).
- The patient vomits and this relieves the headache (K. p. 150: head, pain, vomiting amel.). By vomiting however, the stomach is aggravated so that they will go on vomiting (K. p. 510: nausea, vomiting does not amel.).

SPIGELIA-headache

- The pain is situated on a small spot on the left temple or left side of the face (K. p. 169: head, pain, temples, left; K. p. 217: head, pain, tearing, forehead, eminence, frontal, left).
- The patient indicates the pain with 1 finger (K. p. 148: head, pain, spot, pain in small).
- The pain always remains in the same place (d.d. KALI-BI.: the pain removes).

BRYONIA-headache

- The pain begins on the left of the forehead, mostly above the left eye (K. P. 159: head, pain, forehead, eyes, above left), then extends all over the head and afterwards to the whole body so that all muscles are painful (K. p. 160: head, pain, forehead, eyes, above left, extending to occiput and finally over whole body).
- The patient lies very still, because every motion causes more pain (K. p. 143: head, pain, motion, from).
- Even a movement of the eyes makes the headache worse (K. p. 144: head, pain, moving eyes; moving eyelids).

PULSATILLA-headache

- The headache occurs especially during the menopause in women (K. p. 143: head, pain, menses, during, suppressed; menses, after, cessation, on).
- The headache is worse in warmth and in the sun (K. p. 149: head, pain, sun, from exposure to; K. p. 151: head, pain, warm room).
- The headache is ameliorated in open air and by cold applications (K. p. 136: head, pain, air, open, amel.; K. p. 138: head, pain, cold applications amel.).

STAPHYSAGRIA-headache

- Is an important remedy for headaches.
- The headache starts after a quarrel or a confrontation (K. p. 139: head, pain, excitement of the emotions, after).
- The headache begins after VEXATION or after suppressed anger (K. p. 150: head, pain, vexation, after; K. p. 136: head, pain, anger, from).

MERCURIUS SOLUBILIS–headache

- They have a pain in the form of a band round the head as if the patient wore a helmet (K. p. 189: head, pain, pressing, band, as if by).
- There is <u>salivation</u> during the headache (K. p. 418: mouth, salivation, headache, during).

PAPER CASE : MENYANTHES

Vassilis comes up with a paper case. It is about a case with a HEADACHE. Via the headache, there are no clear keynotes and no remedy is clearly indicated. Via the constitution, there is information available for at least 10 polychrests, but for every polychrest, there are some negative points, so no remedy is clearly indicated.

The only information that comes up in this case, that is strange and yet very strong is the THIRSTLESSNESS. This will be the only keynote of the case because this symptom was underlined 4 times.

Vassilis proceded as follows: he took the rubric "thirstless" (K. p. 530: stomach, thirstless). He run through all remedies 3rd degree because the remedy had to be among them, said Vassilis. No single remedy seemed to fit with the patient. Because the remedy MENY. was also mentioned 3rd degree in this rubric, he read BOERICKE (p. 430) and saw that it was a headache-remedy, and that the description in Boericke corresponded with the patient's story:

- The headache was better with pressure: the patient pushed his head hard into the pillow.
- Icecold hands and feet.
- Never thirsty.

He gave the patient MENY. 30 and the patient had been without a headache for 3 years and had felt well on every plane.

After 3 years, the patient fell back. Vassilis repeated MENY. 30 (a higher potency wasn't available) and now, the patient has been well for more than 3 years.

PAPER CASE : SILICA

- The case concerns a 39-year-old woman, a student in homœopathy.
- Her main problem is forgetfulness and problems with mental work. She forgets words while speaking or writing. She has difficulties with speaking and writing together. Mental work gives her a headache and exhaustion. She reads very slowly.
- She has severe stage fright, with icecold hands, perspiring and trembling. Also anticipation.
- She is easily frightened, she is very shy. As a child, she was afraid of men. She is unsure, afraid of responsibility. She is slow in everything. Her state of mind changes a lot.
- She is very sensitive to everything that happens round her. She takes over the behaviour of others without their ideas.
- Her sexual energy has decreased seriously.
- She has a serious loss of hair.
- She is chilly, has very cold feet, feels well in warmth and can't bear cold wind +++. Yet, she can't bear heat on her head.
- Physical effort gives her palpitations and makes her perspire.
- She has little thirst, likes tea.
- She likes bread and butter, sweet and sour.
- She doesn't like sour fruit or sour drinks.
- She has abundant menses and yellow leucorrhoea.
- She can't fall asleep easily and is never wide awake in the morning.

DISCUSSION BY VASSILIS

- There is a possibility for BARYTA CARBONICA because of the bad memory, the difficulties with taking responsibility, anticipation, chilliness and the loss of hair.

- The majority of symptoms however fit well with <u>SILICA</u>: we see a general weakness: <u>not enough stamina on all levels</u>:

    - stage fright, shyness, anticipation.
    - worse in the winter and with a draft of air.
    - easily frightened: 1st remedy is SIL.
    - sensitive to the position of the moon (full moon, half moon or other positions). Sensitive to the environment.
    - possible fear of everything.
    - loss of hair.
    - they like refined, soft work.

```
┌─────────────────────────────────────────────────────────┐
│                                                           │
│                        TIPS                               │
│                                                           │
│                                                           │
└─────────────────────────────────────────────────────────┘
```

Here, you will find some information that has been gathered in the
course of this seminar.

- Think of DROSERA with the triad:
              - cough after midnight
              - nose bleeding
              - whooping cough

- In case of trembling from cold, think of RHUS-T. and HEP.

- In case of trembling from weakness, think of GELS.

- When there is a clear swelling of the glands in the neck with hard
  painful glands together with a swelling of the glands in the
  armpits and a diminished sense of hearing because of an
  obstruction of the Eustachian tube (the patient can't understand
  you), think of following remedies (K. p. 394):

  1. BARYTA MURIATICA:
     When the patient is chilly. Think of BAR-M. rather than of
     BAR-C. in acute diseases.

2. BROMIUM:
If the patient is warm blooded. BROM. can also be used in acute cases.

3. MERCURIUS SOLUBILIS:
In case of salivation during sleep and offensive breath.

- When a child shows all the symptoms of PULS. but the worst troubles are at night between 2 and 4 a.m., think of KALI-S.

- Epilepsy after trauma of the head, in order of importance:

  1. NAT-S.
  2. CUPR.
  3. HYPER.
  4. ARN.
  5. CIC.

- Strongest remedies for photophobia are: 1. BELL.
  2. GRAPH.
  3. NAT-S.

- Photomania = STRAM.: they are irritable, anxious or depressed when they see the reflexion of light in a mirror or on water.

- In an acute disease, GELS. can also have photophobia and as widely dilated pupils as BELL.

- RATANHIA is a common remedy for haemorrhoids. The patient has a pain as if there is broken glass in the rectum.

- Stomach, pain, night, 2 a.m. (K. p. 512): in order of importance:
  1. KALI-C.
  2. ARS.
  3. LYC.
  4. MED.

MED. is mostly better at night, they are night-people.

- POTHOS.: the asthma is better after stool.

- CARB-V.: is always better with eructations. Even the asthma (K. p. 765 and 769) and the oppression (K. p. 839) or heart palpitations (K. p. 875) are better then.

- Afternoon, sleep, agg. (K. p. 1402):

    1. STAPH.: is psychologically worse afterwards.
    2. SULPH.: will have a burning stomach and sour eructations afterwards.
    3. BRY.: has a feeling as if there is a stone in the stomach.

- ARS. is always chilly, and yet may have a warm head.

- ANTIMONIUM CRUDUM sometimes have a snow-white furred tongue. ANT-C. is aggravated by wine. It is a remedy with an aggravation in the summer. It can be used for hiccough.

- Vomiting in children: 1. IP.: if the tongue is not furred.
    2. SIL.
    3. AETH.: when they are sleepy after vomiting.

- When a child shrieks before or during urination and at the same time reaches for his genitalia, you have to think of ACON., especially when the child is anxious and in a panic.

- Constipation in children who have a hard stool and weep in advance because they know making stool will hurt, makes you think of NUX-V., especially if they are irritable and have a continuous urge to make stool while nothing comes.

- CLEMATIS ERECTA can be used for stenosis of the urethra (even iatrogenic) and for prostatic enlargement.

- In case of prostate cancer, think of CONIUM MACULATUM.

- Paralysis of the bladder in older people: think of ARS.

- Problems with dentition in children: in order of importance:

  1. CHAM.
  2. RHEUM.
  3. CALC.
  4. SIL.

- SELFISH, EGOTISM:
  - PLAT.: vain, they feel they are the best, they look down on all women on the earth.
  - IGN.: thinks that the others are stupid, they are smart and competent.
  - SULPH.: see: essence.

- The combination "offensive perspiring feet + skin eruptions + extreme chilliness" makes you think of GRAPH.

- The most important remedies with erotic dreams are STAPH. and NAT-P.

- Remedies with a desire for salt:
  - desire salt as strong as desire fat with a chilly person makes you think of NIT-AC.
  - desire fat, desire salt, desire sweets, desire sour makes you think of MED.
  - desire salt as strong as desire sour, both very strong, makes you think of VERAT.

- In case of an apparent PULS. who weeps, is sensitive, has menopause complaints, varicose legs, who doesn't like the sun and is thirstless, but has a strong desire for fat: leave PULS. and look for another remedy.

- With an apparent NAT-M. who likes fat: leave NAT-M. and look for another remedy.

- ALOE. is dry around the anus and is ameliorated by cold applications.
  SULPH. is moist around the anus and is aggravated by washing or bathing.

- <u>Cracks in the skin</u> as if being cut with a knife, and which are dry: think of NIT-AC. if they like fat and of PETR. if they dislike fat.

- <u>COLCHICUM</u>: is irritable, has stomach or intestinal problems and can't stand the odor of food, especially of eggs and fish. It makes them feel nauseated or they can faint.

- Remedies who suffer from exposure to the <u>sun</u>, in order of priority:
  1. NAT-C.
  2. GLON.
  3. NAT-M.
  4. PULS.
  5. SULPH.

- Think of GRAPH. in case of skin eruptions with a <u>honey-like discharge</u>. If the discharge is much thicker than honey, so that you can pluck it with a finger, think of KALI-BI.

- Fear of high places as a symptom can decrease, but will mostly not disappear completely.

- <u>Allergy to cow's milk</u> in children: think firstly of TUB.

- <u>Aversion milk</u>: especially think of NIT-AC. and NAT-C.

- <u>Allergic rhinitis with itching eyes</u> which is better from cold water in the face and with sneezing by which the patient loses urine: think of PULS. in a warm-blooded person and of CAUST. in a chilly person (to be added on K. p. 885).

- In case of <u>scraping posterios nares</u>, add MED. 3rd degree on K. p. 349.

- LAUGHING: - STRAM. laughs very loudly
   - BELL.: red face - angry
   - CANN-I.: laughs continuously, won't stop laughing
   - HYOS.: uses dirty language and laughs childishly.

- LACH. sometimes has red spots on the external throat while they are speaking.

- Important remedies for PSORIASIS.

   1. IRIS VERSICOLOR
      - most important skin disease is psoriasis.
      - in case of a headache, they have decreased sight before or during the headache. The patient may be afraid of becoming blind.

   2. STAPHYSAGRIA
      - According to Vassilis, STAPH. is the best remedy for psoriasis, if there are no deep psychological or mental problems.

- ALOPECIA AREATA: loss of hair in patches. If this occurs after grief, think of PH-AC. or of IGN. If these remedies are not appropriate or if there is no clear constitutional remedy, think of BACILLINUM.

- Desire olives: add LYC. 3rd degree, CALC. and SULPH. 1st degree.
   Aversion olives: add SULPH. 2nd degree.

- In case of itching that is aggravated by perspiration, think of MANGANUM.

- Think of FLUORICUM ACIDUM in case of sexual excess in old people with loss of hair.

- MERC. mostly perspires extensively and the perspiration does not give relief, on the contrary.

- KALI-I.: develops a headache in the morning at 5 a.m. (K. p. 135). They are aggravated by warmth and the sun. They also show the general aggravation of every KALI.: between 2 and 4 a.m.

- Insect bites which cause a strong reaction:
  - after a bee sting, give APIS.
  - after a mosquito bite, give LED.
  - all animal bites: give LED.
  - after bites from sea animals, give LED.

- With retired people who have problems with thinking, who get depressed and want to die because they think nobody needs them: think of AURUM.

- In case of a rhinomeningocoele fistel after a skull injury, think of NAT-S. Vassilis once saw a rhinomeningocoele which closed spontaneously after NAT-S.

- RAPHANUS: the sphere of action of RAPH. is a combination of increased sexual energy and colitis. The colitis causes a sharp pain in the left side of the abdomen with the feeling that there is gas in the abdomen which can't come out (e.g. in the sigmoid or in the descending colon).

- The remedies with the strongest anticipation are: ARG-N., GELS. and LYC.

- Allergy to horses: think of CASTOR EQUI.

- CHINA OFFICINALIS remains very faithful to the doctor. They always come back to you with the message that they are not better. However, they will tell others that you are the best doctor.

- THUNDERSTORM: worst fear is for PHOS. The fear of NAT-C. is stronger than the fear of NAT-M.
  NAT-C. sometimes knows a general aggravation before and mostly during the storm: when the atmoshere changes.
  RHOD. has an aggravation of his joint complaints just before the thunderstorm arrives.

- MED. is generally better at the seaside, both physically and psychologically. If they are angry, they sometimes drive to the seaside, take a walk on the beach and afterwards, they feel much better.

- Have a strong aversion to slimy food: NAT-M., MED. and CALC

- When someone has a shock and is very anxious right after an accident, give ACON.
  If the situation is very serious, with extensive haematoma, give ARN.
  If the patient is in coma and breathes in a snoring way, think of OPIUM.

INDEX

- (...)   = 0 to 3 lines
- not underlined   = 4 to 10 lines
- bold   = more than 10 lines
- bold + underlined = more than 1 page or Essence

ARUND.	: (A.126)
ASAF.	: (A.15)
AUR.	: (A.14), (A.15), (A.22), (A.35), (A.37), A.42, (A.97), (A.158), (A.177)
AUR-M-N.	: A.158
BACILLINUM	: A.176
BAPT.	: A.115
BAR-C.	: (A.16), (A.48), (A.57), (A.170)
BAR-M.	: A.50, A.57, (A.171)
BELL.	: (A.26), (A.52), (A.55), A.58, **A.60**, A.65, A.137, **A.163**, (A.165), (A.172), (A.176)
BERB.	: (A.82)
BISM.	: (A.66)
BOR.	: (A.106)
BROM.	: (A.172)
BRY.	: (A.34), (A.44), (A.48), (A.53), A.63, **A.72**, (A.82), (A.85), (A.93), A.166, (A.173)
CALC.	: (A.27), (A.31), A.68, A.114, **A.129**, (A.141), (A.174), (A.176), (A.178)
CALC-AR.	: A.141
CALC-S.	: (A.113), (A.117), (A.134), (A.138), A.142
CALC-SIL.	: A.140
CAMPH.	: (A.84), A.88, A.91, (A.93)
CANN-I.	: (A.49), (A.176)
CANTH.	: **A.78**, (A.81)
CARB-V.	: A.74, A.90, (A.92), (A.173)
CAST.	: (A.177)
CAUST.	: **A.45**, (A.52), (A.62), (A.72), (A.139), (A.151), (A.152), (A.162), (A.175)
CHAM.	: (A.71), A.119, (A.174)
CHEL.	: A.43, **A.69**, (A.71)
CHIN.	: A.43, (A.177)
CIC.	: (A.172)
CLEM.	: (A.81), (A.173)
COC-C.	: A.62
COLCH.	: (A.175)
COLOC.	: (A.18), **A.72**, (A.90), A.91, (A.93)
CON.	: **A.154**, (A.173)
CROT-T.	: **A.89**
CUPR.	: (A.45), A.61, **A.85**, (A.93), (A.120), (A.172)
DIOS.	: **A.71**, (A.73)
DROS.	: **A.61**, (A.171)

DULC.	: (A.52), (A.85), (A.86), (A.88), A.93
ELAPS.	: A.69
EQUIS.	: A.80
EUPHR.	: **A.125**, (A.126)
EUP-PER.	: **A.44**
FERR-P.	: A.45
FL-AC.	: (A.176)
GAMB.	: (A.87), A.89
GELS.	: (A.16), **A.48**, (A.106), (A.163), A.164, (A.171), (A.172), (A.177)
GLON.	: (A.54), (A.175)
GRAPH.	: (A.14), (A.34), **A.71, A.132, A.134**, (A.172), (A.174), (A.175)
HELL.	: **A.150**, (A.151), **A.152**
HEP.	: **A.47**, A.57, (A.59), (A.138), A.142, (A.171)
HYOS.	: (A.22), (A.51), (A.87), (A.176)
HYPER.	: (A.172)
IGN.	: (A.9), (A.16), (A.17), (A.18), (A.33), (A.36), (A.72), (A.102), (A.105), (A.155), (A.174), (A.176)
IOD.	: (A.27)
IP.	: A.62, A.73, (A.173)
IRIS.	: A.164, A.176
KALI-AR.	: (A.21)
KALI-BI.	: A.52, (A.127), (A.165), (A.175)
KALI-C.	: (A.46), (A.64), **A.66**, (A.89), (A.104), (A.172)
KALI-I.	: (A.133), (A.177)
KALI-M.	: (A.64)
KALI-S.	: (A.64), (A.172)
LACH.	: (A.22), (A.48), (A.55), A.56, (A.123), A.142, A.162, (A.176)
LED.	: A.137, A.177
LEM-M.	: A.128
LIL-T.	: (A.15)
LOB.	: A.75
LYC.	: (A.33), (A.46), (A.50), (A.55), (A.56), (A.57), (A.68), **A.70**, (A.104), (A.110), (A.139), (A.153), (A.172), (A.176), (A.177)
MAG-C.	: **A.118**
MAG-M.	: (A.119), (A.120)
MAG-P.	: (A.68), A.90, A.119

PULS.	: (A.18), (A.27), A.32, (A.45), (A.46), (A.50), **A.51**, (A.63), **A.73**, (A.79), (A.90), A.92, (A.102), (A.105), (A.111), (A.114), (A.123), (A.125), (A.130), (A.133), (A.139), (A.148), A.166, (A.172), (A.174), (A.175)
PYROG.	: A.115
RAN-B.	: (A.52), A.63, (A.68)
RAPH.	: A.177
RAT.	: (A.172)
RHEUM.	: A.91, (A.174)
RHOD.	: (A.177)
RHUS-T.	: (A.28), (A.44), **A.49**, (A.52), (A.53), (A.82), A.88, (A.114), A.135, (A.171)
RHUS-V.	: A.135
RUMX.	: A.48, (A.64)
SABAD.	: **A.126**
SANG.	: A.74, A.165
SARS.	: **A.76**, (A.78), (A.81), (A.82), (A.135), (A.139)
SEP.	: (A.18), (A.27), (A.29), **A.30**, (A.33), (A.40), (A.45), (A.51), (A.52), **A.79**, A.157
SIL.	: (A.18), A.138, A.141, (A.142), (A.155), A.157, (A.163), A.169, A.170, (A.173), (A.174)
SIN-N.	: A.126
SPIG.	: A.165
SPONG.	: A.47, (A.51), (A.62)
SQUIL.	: (A.45)
STANN.	: (A.64)
STAPH.	: (A.19), (A.72), (A.76), A.81, (A.102), A.166, (A.173), (A.174), (A.176)
STICT.	: A.127
STRAM.	: (A21), (A.172), (A.176)
SULPH.	: (A.21), (A.28), (A.42), **A.50**, (A.52), (A.53), (A.64), A.70, (A.84), **A.86**, A.87, (A.89), **A.94**, (A.99), **A.116**, (A.125), A.137, (A.139), (A.148), (A.173), (A.174), (A.175), (A.176)
SYMPH.	: (A.21)
SYPH.	: (A.98)
TARENT.	: (A.14)
TELL.	: (A.104)
TER.	: A.81
TEUCR.	: A.127
THEA.	: (A.99)

THUJ.	: A.42, (A.106)
TUB.	: (A.108), (A.175)
URT-U.	: A.136
UVA.	: A.80
VERAT.	: (A.21), (A.27), (A.31), (A.66), **A.84**, (A.85), (A.93), (A.174)
WYE.	: A.54, **A.123**
ZINC.	: A.151

Do you want to be informed about the books of Dr. Med.
Vassilis GHEGAS which will be published soon?

Please send your name and address to:

HOMEO-STUDY v.z.w.
De Schom 67, B-3600 GENK
BELGIUM

The following Dutch seminars of Vassilis GHEGAS will soon be translated in English:

November 1987 — Essences: IGN., NAT-C., NAT-P.
— Essences: NIT-AC., SUL-AC., FL-AC.,
LAC-AC., ACET-AC., BENZ-AC.

April 1988 — Essences: SIL., PH-AC., PIC-AC.
— Newborns, babies and children.
— Types of children: STRAM., HYOS., CHAM.,
MED.

November 1988 — Essences: SEP., MUR-AC., STAPH.
— Types of children: MED., VERAT., HYOS.,
CAUST., STAPH., NAT-M., NAT-S., IOD., CI-
NA., LACH., CALC., CALC-P., TUB.

April 1989 — Essences: ARS., PETR., PLB., RAN-B.
— Types of children: MANC., AUR., SULPH.,
PHOS., PULS., CHAM., RHEUM., BAR-C.,
GRAPH., IOD., CHIN.
— Skin disorders.

1987 - 1989 — How to take the case.
How to handle the patient.

May 1989 — Fears and Phobia
— Essences: FERR., RHUS-T., CALC-S., LAC-C.,
ALUM., CALC-P.

October 1989 — Hyper- and hyposexual remedies.
— Personal development of the patient.
— Philosophy: How does Homœopathy work?

November 1989 — Asthma.
— Complementary remedies.
— D.D. polychrests.
— Remedies in vertigo, hepatitis.

March 1990
- Forgetfulness - remedies.
- Traumata in homœopathy.
- Homœopathy during pregnancy.
- Essences: KALI-C., LACH., TUB.

1984 - 1985
- Essences: SANG., BRY., CHIN., AGAR., IOD., CAUST.
- Remedies in asthma, headache, nose troubles, sciatica, psychiatry, haemorrhoids.
- Philosophy: How does Homœopathy work - the sleep.

1986 - 1988
- Essences: BELL., MED., CON.
- Remedies in gonorrhœa, masturbation, impotence, metrorrhagia.
- Sensitivity graduation of remedies.
- Difficult pathology, cancer, special diseases.

October 1990
- Essences: NUX-V., ANAC., CON., CIMIC.
- Tips for follow-up on the long term and obstructed cases.
- Remedies in trigeminus-neuralgia, leucorrhœa, PSH.
- Epilepsy in children.